Paleo Diet Recipes 365 Days of Paleo
Mercedes Del R(
DOWNLOAD YOUR FREE PALEO EPI

AND START LOSING WEIG

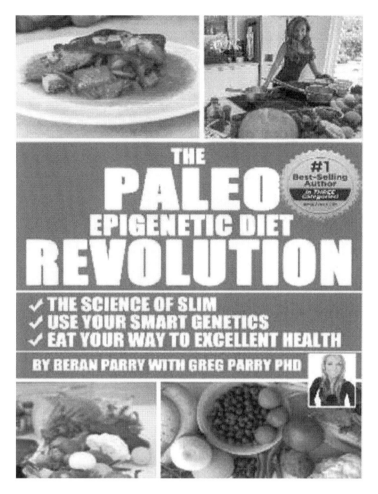

Please search this page over the internet
www.skinnydeliciouslife.com/free-epigenetic-diet-ebook

Paleo Diet Recipes 365 Days of Paleo and Coconut Recipes by Mercedes Del Rey

Paleo Diet Recipes

365 Days

of

Paleo and Coconut Recipes

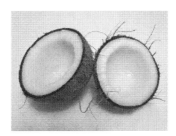

by

Mercedes Del Rey

Paleo Diet Recipes 365 Days of Paleo and Coconut Recipes by Mercedes Del Rey

Copyright © 2017 by Beran Parry

All rights reserved. No part of this publication may be reproduced, distributed, or transmitted in any form or by any means, including photocopying, recording, or other electronic or mechanical methods, without the prior written permission of the publisher, except in the case of brief quotations embodied in critical reviews and certain other non-commercial uses permitted by copyright law. For permission requests, write to the publishers' email address: beranparry@gmail.com

Paleo Diet Recipes 365 Days of Paleo and Coconut Recipes by Mercedes Del Rey
SPECIAL FREE GIFT FROM THE PUBLISHER

The PERFECT PALEO RECIPE BUNDLE
4 Life Changing Books
By Beran Parry

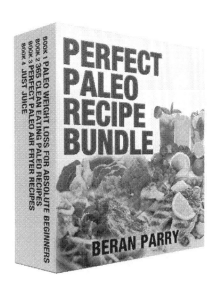

Please search this page over the internet

app.getresponse.com/site2/perfectpaleorecipesbundle?u=mZLi&webforms_id=8541901

Paleo Diet Recipes 365 Days of Paleo and Coconut Recipes by Mercedes Del Rey

FOR MORE BY

MERCEDES DEL REY

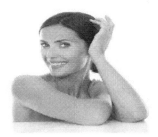

Please search this page over the www.amazon.com
amzn.to/2kSzZnU

Paleo Diet Recipes 365 Days of Paleo and Coconut Recipes by Mercedes Del Rey

INTRODUCTION

Welcome to my world of holistic healing and totally delicious nutrition. My name is Mercedes del Rey but my friends just call me Merche and I am truly fortunate to live in one of the most beautiful places in the world. My home is in the sun-kissed paradise of Andalusia in southern Spain where I am busily planning my holistic wellbeing and nutritional healing centre. This is where I grew up, went to school, studied and graduated before travelling to the US to further my education. My travels and studies have taken me to China and India, Africa and South East Asia and I feel at home wherever I go. I feel I have become what my parents encouraged me to be - a citizen of the world. My purpose in life is to help people to experience the full potential of their wellbeing and I've been guiding and advising individuals on the merits of natural, intelligent nutrition for most of my working life. I want to share my knowledge and experience with you and make a positive difference to the quality of your life

I'm delighted that you have chosen this book full of delicious recipes and hope that you enjoy them all

Paleo Diet Recipes 365 Days of Paleo and Coconut Recipes by Mercedes Del Rey

Contents

INTRODUCTION	7
1. High Protein Breakfast Gold	18
2. Apple Breakfast Dream	19
3. Divine Protein Muesli	20
4. Ultimate Skinny Granola	21
5. Apple Chia Delight	22
6. Chocco Granola Recipe	23
7. Choco Nut Skinny Muesli Balls	24
8. Sweetie Skinny Crackers	25
9. Gutsy Granola	26
10. Breakfast Mexicana	27
11. Paleo Maple-Nut Porridge with Banana	28
12. Raisin Nut Crunch Cereal	29
13. Apple Cider Paleo Donuts	30
14. Prosciutto-Wrapped Mini Frittata Muffins	31
15. Tasty Apple Almond Coconut Medley	32
16. Paleo Garlic Breadsticks (Just Don't Eat Them All Yourself)	33
17. Breakfast Quiche with Broccoli and Ham	34
18. Sun-Dried Tomato Quiche	35
19. Paleo Breakfast Burritos (Low-Carb)	36
20. Bake Eggs in the Oven	37
21. Baked Eggs in Ham Cups	38
22. Grain-Free "French Toast" Breakfast Chalupa	39
23. Paleo Sausage Balls	40
24. Macadamia Mix Breakfast	41
25. Cherry Almond Muesli Recipe	42
26. Macadamia Mix Breakfast	43
27. Chocco Granola Recipe	44
28. Cherry Almond Muesli Recipe	45
29. Vegetarian Curry with Squash	46
30. Spectacular Spaghetti and Delish Turkey Balls	47
31. Sensational Courgette Pasta and Turkey Bolognaise	48
32. Ostrich Steak or Venison with Divine Mustard Sauce and Roasted Tomatoes	49
33. Tantalizing Turkey Pepper Stir-fry	50
34. Cheeky Chicken Stir Fry	51
35. Chicken Fennel Stir-Fry	52
36. Muddy Buddy Recipe	53

Paleo Diet Recipes 365 Days of Paleo and Coconut Recipes by Mercedes Del Rey

37. Creamy Chicken Casserole 54
38. Vegetarian Curry with Squash 55
39. Red Cabbage Bonanza Salad 56
40. Paleo Crock Pot Cashew Chicken 57
41. Spicy Slow Cooker Chorizo Chili 58
42. Crock-Pot Roast 59
43. Paleo Mini Meatloaves 60
44. Kale and Red Pepper Frittata 61
45. The Best Homemade Ranch Dressing Ever 62
47. Easy Paleo Slow Cooker Pot Roast 64
48. Red Cabbage Bonanza Salad 65
49. Sausage and Kale "Pasta" Casserole 66
50. Divine Chicken or Turkey and Baby Bok Choy Salad 67
51. Broiled Curry Coconut Sole or Cod 68
52. Sexy Shrimp on Sticks 69
53. Delicious Fish Stir Fry 70
54. Spectacular Salmon 71
55. Creamy Coconut Salmon 72
56. Salmon Dill Bonanza 73
57. Sexy Shrimp Cocktail 74
58. Gambas al Ajillo--Sizzling Garlic Shrimp 75
59. Spicy Granola 76
60. Scrambled Eggs with Chilli 77
61. Spicy India Omelet 78
62. Mushrooms, Eggs and Onion Bonanza 79
63. Spicy Turkey Stir Fry 80
64. Turkey and Kale Pasta Casserole 81
65. Roasted and Filled Tasty Bell Peppers 82
66. Creamy Chicken Casserole 83
67. Spectacular Spaghetti and Delish Turkey Balls 84
68. Sensational Courgette Pasta and Turkey Bolognaise 85
69. Perfect Turkey Stir-Fry 86
70. Creamy Curry Stir Fry 87
71. Chicken Coconut Divine 88
72. Coconut Turkey Salad 89
73. Jolly Jamaican Chicken 90
74. Thai Baked Fish with Squash Noodles 91
75. Divine Prawn Mexicana 92
76. Shrimp Cakes Delux 93

Paleo Diet Recipes 365 Days of Paleo and Coconut Recipes by Mercedes Del Rey

77. Shrimp Spinach Spectacular 94
78. Turkey Eastern Surprise 95
79. Spaghetti Squash Hash Browns 96
80. Super Tempting Tofu 97
81. Crispy Baked Chicken Fingers 98
82. Balsamic Glaze Chicken Wings 99
83. Zucchini Fritters 100
84. Sundried Tomato Roulade 101
85. Beefy Shanky Broth 102
86. Coconut Crusted Baked Cauliflower Bites 103
87. Crockpot Maple and Balsamic Glazed pork Loin 104
88. Cauliflower Buffalo Bites 105
89. Spicy Steak 106
90. Dark Chocolate 107
91. Totally Tahini Cups 108
92. Pumpkin crepes 109
93. Lemon Cookies 110
94. Banana Shake 111
95. Spectacular Spinach Omelet 112
96. Blushing Blueberry Omelet 113
97. Roasted and Filled Tasty Bell Peppers 114
98. Creamy Chicken Casserole 115
99. Ostrich Steak or Venison with Divine Mustard Sauce and Roasted Tomatoes 116
100. Tantalizing Turkey Pepper Stir-fry 117
101. Cheeky Chicken Stir Fry 118
102. Turkey Thai Basil 119
103. Chicken Fennel Stir-Fry 120
104. Prawn garlic Fried "Rice" 121
105. Lemon and Thyme Super Salmon 122
106. Spectacular Spaghetti and Delish Turkey Balls 123
107. Prawn Salad Boats 124
108. Sexy Shrimp with Delish Veggie Stir Fry 125
109. Peachy Prawn Coconut 126
110. Rosy Chicken Supreme Salad 127
111. Creamy Carrot Salad 128
112. Quick And Easy Broth 129
113. Turkey Stockbroth 130
114. Simple Beef and Broccoli Stir Fry 131
115. Homemade Sweet and Salty Paleo Granola 132

Paleo Diet Recipes 365 Days of Paleo and Coconut Recipes by Mercedes Del Rey

116. Curry Coconut Salad 133
117. Prawn garlic Fried "Rice" 134
118. Creamy Carrot Salad 135
119. Skinny Chicken salad 136
120. Spectacular Spinach Omelet 137
121. Blushing Blueberry Omelet 138
122. Paleo Shrimp Fried "Rice" 139
123. Asparagus Quiche with Spaghetti Squash Crust 140
124. Garden Pea, Feta & Mint Tart 141
125. Garlicky Collard Pie 142
126. Crustless Broccoli and Sausage Quiche 143
127. Bacon and Tomato Quiche 144
128. Paleo Turkey Pesto Meatballs 146
129. Broccoli Egg Bake (So Wholesome & Healthy) 147
130. Meatball Sandwich with Zucchini "Bread" & Coconut Curry Sauce 148
131. Spicy Steak 149
132. Easy Homemade Gluten-Free Energy Bars 150
133. Gummi Orange Slices 151
134. Spicy Steak 152
135. Baked Sweet Potato Chips 153
136. Gummi Orange Slices 154
137. Prosciutto-Wrapped Berries 155
138. Vanilla Pumpkin Seed Clusters 156
139. Almond Joy Sunday 157
140. Spiced Autumn Apples Baked in Brandy 158
141. Chocolate Bavarian Cheesecake 159
142. Maple Cinnamon Cheesecakes with Gingerbread Crust 160
143. Heavenly Raw Vegan White Chocolate and Raspberry Cheesecake 161
144. Samoa Donuts 162
145. Hummingbird Bread 164
146. Earl Grey Lavender Ice Cream 165
147. Blueberry Cream Pie 166
148. Gluten Free Dairy Free Coconut 167
149. Grain Free Steamed Christmas Puddings – GAPS & Paleo Friendly 168
150. Raw Pineapple Coconut Vegan Cheesecake 169
151. Grain-free Italian Lemon Almond Cake 170
152. Cheeky Cherry Crisp 171
153. Stunning Key Lime Pie 172
154. Delectable Cocoa-Nut Apples 173

Paleo Diet Recipes 365 Days of Paleo and Coconut Recipes by Mercedes Del Rey

- 155. Outstanding Hazelnut Banana 174
- 156. Cookies with Dark Chocolate 175
- 157. Lemon Almond Delight 176
- 158. Ginger Vanilla Extravaganza 177
- 159. Cute Cupcakes Recipe 178
- 160. Strawberry Chessecake Delight 179
- 161. Creative Cardamom Cupcakes 180
- 162. Apple, almond & blackberry Bonanza 181
- 163. Almond Happiness Bars 182
- 164. Sexy Coconut Crack Bars 183
- 165. Lemonny Lemon Delights 184
- 166. Macadamia Pineapple Bonanza 185
- 167. Pretty Pumpkin Delights 186
- 168. Sexy Dessert Pan 187
- 169. Peachy Creamy Peaches 189
- 170. Creamy Berrie Pie 190
- 171. Choco - Coconut Berry Ice 191
- 172. Cheeky Cherry Ice 192
- 173. Creamy Caramely Ice Cream 193
- 174. Berry Ice Cream and Almond Delight 194
- 175. Eastern Spice Delights 195
- 176. Absolute Almond Bites 196
- 177. Choco Coco Cookies 197
- 178. Chococups 198
- 179. Choco – Almond Delights 199
- 180. Fetching Fudge 200
- 181. Nut Butter Truffles 201
- 182. Extra Dark Choco Delight 202
- 183. Chestnut- Cacao Cake 203
- 184. Apple Cinnamon Walnut Bonanza 204
- 185. Choco Triple Delight.. 205
- 186. Choco Cookie Delight 206
- 187. Best Ever Banana Surprise Cake 207
- 188. Coco – Walnut Brownie Bites 208
- 189. Choco-coco Brownies.. 209
- 190. Spectacular Spinach Brownies 210
- 191. Best Banana Nut Bread 211
- 192. Carrot Coconut Surprise 212
- 193. Relishing Raisin Bread 213

Paleo Diet Recipes 365 Days of Paleo and Coconut Recipes by Mercedes Del Rey

194. Luscious Lemon Delight 214
195. Sexy Sweet Potato 215
196. Cheeky Coconut Loaf 216
197. Heavenly Herb Flatbread 217
198. Cozy Coconut Flour Muffins 218
199. Naked Chocolate Cake 219
200. Blueberry Sponge Roll Surprise 220
201. Lemon Mousse Mouthwatering Cupcakes 221
202. Chocolate Raspberry Cake Delight 222
203. Strawberry Dashing Doughnuts 223
204. Perfect Plantain Cake Surprise 224
205. Lemon Blueberry Cake Delight 225
206. Delicious Coconut Flour Cake with Strawberry Surprise 226
207. Titillating Berry Trifle 227
208. Lemon-Coconut Petit Fours 229
209. Gingerbread Cream Delight 230
210. Mouthwatering Coconut Custard Cake 231
211. Cranberry Orange Upside Down Revolution 232
212. Baked Vanilla Cardamom Delights 233
213. Pumpkin Cream Cookies 234
214. Sexy Savory Muffins 235
215. Delicious Lady Fingers 236
216. Cheeky Coconut Chocolate Cookies 237
217. Scrumptious Peanut Butter Parcels 238
218. Chocolaty Pumpkin Muffins 239
219. Succulent Shortbread Cookies 240
220. Tasty Coconut Pancakes 241
221. Fluffy Coconut Flour Waffles 242
222. Sexy Savory Pannukakku 242
223. Fudgy Coconut Flour Brownies 243
224. Delectable Pumpkin Bars 244
225. Mouthwatering Lemon Bars 245
226. Yummy Pumpkin Bars 246
227. Delicious Coconut Biscuits 247
228. Beautiful Butternut Pitta Surprise 248
229. Onion Herb Coconut Biscuits 249
230. Oniony Delishy Biscuits 250
231. Crisp Coconut Flour Tortillas 251
232. Easy Delish Pizza Crust Recipe 252

Paleo Diet Recipes 365 Days of Paleo and Coconut Recipes by Mercedes Del Rey

233. Coconut Pretty Pizza Crust 253
234. Creamy Appetizing Croissant 254
235. Delicious Gnocchi Balls 255
236. Crispy Coconut Crackers 256
237. Tempting Custard Pie 257
238. Nutritious Paleo Tortillas 258
239. Luscious Chocolate-Caramel Brownies 259
240. Fudgy Pumpkin Blondies 260
241. Spinach Brownies Revisited 261
242. Celebratory Chocolate Hazelnut Cupcakes 262
243. Bursting Banana Cupcakes (nut-free) with Whipped White Chocolate Sesame Frosting ...263
244. Lovely Lemon Cupcakes with Lemon Frosting (2 Variations)(Nut-Free) 264
245. Sexy Red Velvet Chocolate Cupcakes With Coconut-Cherry Glaze 265
246. Party Pink Velvet Cupcakes with Vanilla Frosting 266
247. Chocolate Cupcakes with Coconut Cream Filling 267
248. Delish Apple Pie Cupcakes with Cinnamon Frosting 268
249. Pumpkin Coco Cupcakes with creamy cinnamon filling 269
250. Bursting Banana Choco Cupcakes 270
251. Jam and 'Cream' Cupcakes 271
252. Delicious Yellow Cupcake Recipe 272
253. Perfect Pear & Nutmeg Cupcakes 273
254. Xmas Chocolate Chip Cupcakes 274
255. Boston Cream Pie Cupcake Bonanza 275
256. Vanilla Bean Cupcakes with Mocha Buttercream 277
257. Meaty Meatloaf Cupcakes 278
258. Gushing Guava Cupcakes with Whipped Guava Frosting 279
259. Blushing Blueberry Muffin Recipe 281
260. Healthy Carrot Ginger Muffins 282
261. Pecan Muffins 283
262. Temptingly Perfect Plantain Drop 284
263. Sweety Potato Muffins 285
264. Zesty Zucchini Muffins 286
265. Cozy Coconut Flour Muffins 287
266. Lemon Mousse Mouthwatering Cupcakes 288
267. Sexy Savory Muffins 289
268. Molten Lava Chocolate Cupcake 290
269. Party Carrot Cupcakes 291
270. Cinnamon Chocolate Chip Muffins 292
271. Strawberry Shortcake Cupcakes 293

Paleo Diet Recipes 365 Days of Paleo and Coconut Recipes by Mercedes Del Rey

- 272. Thin Mint Mini Cupcakes 294
- 273. Lemon-Coconut Petit Fours 295
- 274. Blushing Blueberry Cupcakes 296
- 275. Delicious Morning Cupcakes 297
- 276. Cheerful Coffee Cupcake 298
- 277. Luscious Lemon Poppy Seed Cupcake 299
- 278. Strawberry chia Cupcake 300
- 279. Triple Coconut Cupcakes 301
- 280. Lemon-Coconut Muffins 302
- 281. Chocolate Banana Muffins 303
- 282. Delicious English Cupcakes 304
- 283. Amazing Almond Flour Cupcakes 305
- 284. Delightful Cinnamon Apple Muffins 306
- 285. Delish Banana Nut Muffins 307
- 286. Apple Cinnamon Muffins 308
- 287. Apple Cardamom Cupcakes 309
- 288. Chocolate Olive Oil Cupcakes 310
- 289. One-Bowl Coconut Flour Cupcakes 312
- 290. Meatloaf Cupcakes 313
- 291. Gluten Free Banana Nut Bread 314
- 292. Pumpkin crepes 315
- 293. Red Coconut Smoothie 316
- 294. Briana's House Low Carb Chocolate Chip Cookies 317
- 295. Coconut Vanilla Surprise 318
- 296. Tempting Coconut Berry Smoothie 319
- 297. Pineapple Coconut Deluxe Smoothie 320
- 298. Sumptuous Strawberry Coconut Smoothie 321
- 299. Divine Peach Coconut Smoothie 322
- 300. Raspberry Coconut Smoothie 323
- 301. Sweet Melon 324
- 302. CINNAMON Coconut Surprise 325
- 303. Low Carb Fried Zucchini 326
- 304. Slow Cooker Paleo Mexican Breakfast Casserole 327
- 305. Paleo Pumpkin Pie Smoothie 328
- 306. Paleo Cookie Butter 329
- 307. Paleo-friendly Coconut Chocolate Coffee Cake 331
- 308. Grain Free Steamed Christmas Puddings – GAPS & Paleo Friendly 332
- 309. Paleo Antioxidant Berry Shake 333
- 310. Perfect Paleo Loaf 334

Paleo Diet Recipes 365 Days of Paleo and Coconut Recipes by Mercedes Del Rey

311. Raw Pineapple Coconut Vegan Cheesecake 335
312. Nutritious Paleo Tortillas 336
313. Perfect Paleo Bananacado Fudge Cupcakes 337
314. Paleo Sticky Date Pudding Cupcakes 338
315. Vanilla Paleo Cupcakes 339
316. Paleo Vanilla Cupcakes 340
317. Paleo Chocolate Cupcake with "Peanut Butter" Frosting 341
318. Addictive & Healthy Paleo Nachos 342
319. Homemade Paleo Tortilla Chips 343
320. Paleo Chocolate Cookies (I Can't Get Enough of These) 344
321. Easy Paleo Shepherd's Pie 345
322. Paleo Apple Pie Cupcakes with Cinnamon Frosting 346
323. Paleo French Toast with Blueberry Syrup 347
324. The Best Paleo Brownies (Chocolaty Goodness) 348
325. Paleo Chocolate Cranberry Muffins 349
326. Salt and Vinegar Zucchini Chips 350
327. Nutritious Paleo Tortillas 351
328. Perfect Paleo Bananacado Fudge Cupcakes 352
329. Incredibly Easy Paleo Chicken Soup 353
330. Paleo Chicken Soup 354
331. Paleo Chicken Soup with Nuddles 355
332. PALEO CROCK POT CHICKEN SOUP 356
333. Paleo Stuffed Breakfast Peppers 357
334. Blushing Beet Salad 358
335. Cheeky Chicken Salad 359
336. Melting Mustard Chicken 360
337. Easy Paleo Spaghetti Squash & Meatballs 361
338. Paleo Pulled Pork Sliders 362
339. Basic Balsamic Steak Marinade 363
340. Lemon Tilapia Ajillo 364
341. Paleo crock Bone Broth 365
342. Paleo Phobroth 366
343. Fantastic Paleo Broth 367
344. Tasty Tomato Tilapia 368
345. Beet Sprout Divine Salad 369
346. Paleo Keto Bone Broth 370
347. Faux Paleo Napoleon 371
348. Fish Fillet Delux 372
349. Roasted Paleo Citrus and Herb Chicken 373

Paleo Diet Recipes 365 Days of Paleo and Coconut Recipes by Mercedes Del Rey

- 350. Stove-top "Cheesy" Paleo Chicken Casserole ... 374
- 351. Homemade Herbed Paleo Mayonnaise ... 375
- 352. Homemade Paleo Ketchup with a Kick ... 376
- 353. Homemade Paleo Honey Mustard from Scratch ... 377
- 354. All-Natural Homemade Paleo Apple Butter ... 378
- 355. Homemade Paleo BBQ Sauce (YUM) ... 379
- 356. Basil Pesto ... 380
- 357. Paleo Chicken Tortilla Soup ... 381
- 358. Paleo Eggs Benedict on Artichoke Hearts ... 382
- 359. Hearty Paleo Jambalaya ... 383
- 360. Shrimp & Grits (Paleo Style) ... 384
- 361. How to Make Paleo Cauliflower "Rice" ... 385
- 362. Paleo Cocoa Puffs ... 386
- 363. Tantalizing Prawn Skewers ... 387
- 364. Paleo BLT Frittata ... 388
- 365. Extra Easy Broth ... 389
- About The Author ... 390
- Before You Go....... ... 393

Paleo Diet Recipes 365 Days of Paleo and Coconut Recipes by Mercedes Del Rey

1. High Protein Breakfast Gold

Ingredients:
1/2 c. Flax-Meal, golden
1/2 c. Chia seed
Stevia liquid to taste
2 tbs. dark ground cinnamon
1 tbs. hemp protein powder
2 tbs. coconut oil, melted

1 tsp. vanilla extract 3/4 c. + 2 tbs. hot water
Instructions:
Begin to spread the dough out until its super thin, onto a parchment paper lined cookie sheet. Bake at 325 for 15 minutes, then drop it down to 300 and leave for 30 minutes. Before dropping it, pull out the sheet and cut it using a pizza roller. Put it back into the oven exactly like this, don't separate the pieces. When the 30 minutes are up, pull it out and separate the pieces. Drop the pieces to 200 degrees F for 1 hour. They will be completely dried out at this point. Enjoy with almond milk!

Paleo Diet Recipes 365 Days of Paleo and Coconut Recipes by Mercedes Del Rey

2. Apple Breakfast Dream

Ingredients:
2 C raw walnuts
1 C raw macadamia nuts
2 apples, peeled and diced
1 Tbsp coconut oil
1 Tbsp ground cinnamon
2 C almond milk
1 14 oz can full fat coconut milk

Instructions:
Combine nuts and dates in a food processor until ground into a fine meal, about 1 minute; set aside.
Saute apples over medium heat in coconut oil until lightly browned, about 5 minutes.
Add nut mixture and cinnamon to apples and stir to incorporate, about 1 minute.
Reduce heat to low and add coconut and almond milk.
Stirring occasionally, let mixture cook uncovered until thickened, about 25 minutes.

3. Divine Protein Muesli

Ingredients:
1 cup unsweetened unsulfured coconut flakes
1 tbsp chopped walnuts
1 tbsp raw almonds (~10)
1 tbsp chocolate chips (soy, dairy, and gluten free brand)
1/2 tsp cinnamon (Ceylon)
1 cup unsweetened almond milk
1 scoop hemp protein
Instructions:
In a medium bowl layer coconut flakes, walnuts, almonds, raisins and chocolate chips.
Sprinkle with cinnamon.
Pour cold almond milk over the muesli and eat with a spoon.

4. Ultimate Skinny Granola

Ingredients:
1 cup of unsweetened coconut milk or unsweetened almond milk or kefir
Stevia liquid to taste
1 tspoon of unsalted pecan pieces
1 tspoon of unsalted walnut pieces
1 tspoon of silvered almonds
1 tspoon of unsalted pistachios
1 tspoon of unsalted raw pine nuts
1 tspoon of unsalted, raw sunflower/safflower seeds
1 tspoon of unsalted, raw pumpkin seeds
2 Tbspoons of frozen or fresh berry selection (e.g. blueberries, blackberries, raspberries, strawberries, or other kinds etc)

Instructions:
Put all the nuts & seeds in a breakfast bowl.
If using unsweetened milk, you could optionally add a teaspoon of pure liquid stevia and stir it well in.
Add the berries and milk.
If using frozen berries, wait for 2-3 minutes for them to get warmer.
The berries will now release some color into the milk, making it look really interesting. Enjoy!

5. Apple Chia Delight

Ingredients:
2c organic chia seeds (black or white)
1c organic hemp hearts
1/2 chopped dried organic apples (or other dried fruit of your choice)
2tbsp real cinnamon
1 tsp low sodium salt
optional: 1/2c chopped nuts of your choice
Instructions:
Throw all of this together, mix it up, and store in a jar in a cool dry place. Stevia to taste.

6. Chocco Granola Recipe

Ingredients
1 & 1/2 cup almonds
1 & 1/2 cup other nuts/seeds (or more almonds. I did a combo of pepitas, sunflower seeds and walnuts)
1 cup flax seed meal
1 cup flaked coconut (unsweetened)
Stevia to taste
1/2 tsp salt
1/3 cup Kelapo coconut oil, melted
1 egg
1/2 cup cacao nibs

Instructions
Preheat oven to 300F and line a large rimmed baking sheet with parchment paper.
In the bowl of a food processor, combine almonds and other nuts or seeds. Pulse until mixture resembles coarse crumbs with some bigger pieces in there too.
Transfer to a large bowl and add flax seed meal, flaked coconut, sweetener of choice, and salt. Drizzle with coconut oil and stir to combine.
Add egg, and toss until mixture begins to clump together. Stir in cacao nibs
Spread mixture evenly on prepared baking sheet and bake 20 minutes, stirring frequently.
Remove and let cool.

7. Choco Nut Skinny Muesli Balls

Ingredients:
1 cup of raw almonds
1 Tablespoon of coconut oil
¼ teaspoon low sodium salt
2 Tablespoon Coconut flour
1 egg white
2 Tablespoon plus 1 teaspoon of Cacao powder
¼ cup of pure liquid stevia

Instructions:
First grind the almonds in a food processor or blender until you have a flour.
Add the ground almonds, low sodium salt, coconut flour, egg white, pure liquid stevia and cacao power to a bowl and mix with a spoon until you have a dough.
Either:
a) Place the dough onto a piece of parchment paper. Place a second piece of parchment paper over the top and roll it until it is ¼" thick. With a wet knife, score it into 1" squares. Place the parchment paper on a baking sheet when finished.
Or
b) Take a small pinch of the dough and roll into a ¼ round ball and set on a baking sheet lined with parchment paper.
Turn on your oven and set to 350 degrees and bake for 15 - 18 minutes for cereal balls or bake for 8 to 12 minutes for flat cereal.
Remove from the oven and let cool on the pan.
Top with your favorite milk and enjoy!

8. Sweetie Skinny Crackers

Ingredients:
1 egg
pure liquid stevia to taste
1 Tbspn coconut oil, melted
1.5 cups almond flour
5 cup coconut flour
1 teaspoon cinnamon

Instructions:
Preheat oven to 350°
In a large bowl, whisk together the egg, pure liquid stevia and melted coconut oil
Add the coconut and almond flour and stir to combine.
Give the dough a couple of kneads so it's well incorporated.
Turn the dough onto a piece of parchment paper and flatten a bit with your hands.
Place another piece of parchment on top and roll out with a rolling pin until it's about 1/8 inch thick.
Remove the top piece of parchment and cut the dough into 1/4 inch squares for cereal, and about 2"x3" for crackers
Sprinkle the cinnamon into the dough mixture.
Slide the dough with the bottom parchment paper onto a baking sheet and bake for 15 minutes.
Turn down the oven to 325° and bake for another 10-15 minutes, or until the cereal / crackers are crisp.

9. Gutsy Granola

Ingredients:
1 cup cashews
3/4 cup almonds
1/4 cup pumpkin seeds, shelled
1/4 cup sunflower seeds, shelled
1/2 cup unsweetened coconut flakes
1/4 cup coconut oil
Stevia to taste
1 tsp vanilla
1 tsp low sodium salt

Instructions:
Preheat oven to 300 degrees F. Line a baking sheet with parchment paper. Place the cashews, almonds, coconut flakes and pumpkin seeds into a blender and pulse to break the mixture into smaller pieces.

In a large microwave-safe bowl, melt the coconut oil, vanilla, and stevia together for 40-50 seconds. Add in the mixture from the blender and the sunflower seeds, and stir to coat.

Spread the mixture out onto the baking sheet and cook for 20-25 minutes, stirring once, until the mixture is lightly browned. Remove from heat. Add low sodium salt.

Press the granola mixture together to form a flat, even surface. Cool for about 15 minutes, and then break into chunks.

10. Breakfast Mexicana

Ingredients:
For the tortillas:
2 eggs
2 egg whites
1/2 cup water
4 tsp ground flaxseed
Pinch of low sodium salt
For the filling:
1 avocado, diced
1/4 cup red bell
pepper, finely diced
1/4 cup onion, finely diced
1/4 cup baked cod or other protein
Handful of spinach leaves
1 tsp coconut oil

Instructions:
In a small bowl, whisk together the ingredients for the tortilla. Preheat the oven
Heat a 10-inch non-stick skillet over medium heat and coat well with coconut oil spray.
Pour half of the tortilla mixture into the pan and swirl to evenly distribute.
Using a metal spatula, loosen the edges of the tortilla from the pan.
Cook a couple of minutes until golden brown on the bottom, and then carefully slide the spatula under the tortilla to loosen it from the bottom of the pan. Do not flip yet.
Place the pan under the broiler for 3-4 minutes until the tortilla gets a little bubbly.
Remove the tortilla from the pan, setting on a piece of aluminum foil. Repeat with other half of tortilla mixture.
After the tortillas are done broiling, preheat the oven to 400 degrees F. In a separate small pan, heat the coconut oil over medium heat.
Add the onions and peppers and sauté for 5-8 minutes, until soft. Add the spinach into the pan and wilt.
Place all of the fillings down the center of the tortillas and wrap tightly. Place into the oven for 5-8 minutes to set. It's so delish!

11. Paleo Maple-Nut Porridge with Banana

Ingredients

½ cup soaked pecans (or a mixture of your preferred nuts). I put some in a bowl overnight if I do not have on hand. I have done this with part macadamia nuts, dreamy!
¾ cup boiling water
2 tablespoons coconut butter (please refer to link above on how to easily make your own)
½ very ripe banana (a soaked medjool date would be another great option!)
2 teaspoons real maple syrup
½ teaspoon cinnamon
⅛ teaspoon sea salt (to taste)

Instructions

In a blender, place all the ingredients and blend until smooth and creamy. Mixture will be thin. If you do not have a high powered blender the nuts will need to be soaked and NOT dehydrated.
Place mixture into a small saucepan over medium low heat. Heat gently until thick and creamy. Serve.

12. Raisin Nut Crunch Cereal

Ingredients

1/2 cup sunflower seeds
1/4 cup pumpkin seeds
2 Tbsp. squash seeds (or more pumpkin seeds)
1/2 cup almond meal (I used dried almond pulp from making almond milk)
1 1/3 cup coconut
1 cup almonds, chopped
1 1/2 tsp. cinnamon
3 Tbsp. coconut oil
1/4 cup raw honey
1 tsp. vanilla
1 cup raisins (added after cereal is baked)

Directions

1. Preheat oven to 325 degrees.
2. Combine all dry ingredients (except raisins).
3. Warm coconut oil and honey slightly so they are easily incorporated. Pour oil, honey and vanilla over dry ingredients. Mix well
4. Spread cereal mixture over large baking pan (15 x 10 or bigger) and bake at 325 degrees for 20 minutes. Take out of oven, stir mixture and bake for another 5-7 minutes.
5. Cool. Add raisins and serve with homemade coconut milk or homemade almond milk! Store in an airtight container.

13. Apple Cider Paleo Donuts

Ingredients (makes 10-12 mini-donuts)
Paleo Donuts
1/2 cup coconut flour
1/2 teaspoon cinnamon
1/2 teaspoon baking soda
1/8 teaspoon celtic sea salt
2 eggs (room temperature)
2 tablespoons honey
2 tablespoons coconut oil (liquid)
1/2 cup warm apple cider
2 tablespoons ghee (or butter or coconut oil), melted – for coating cooked donuts
Cinnamon Sugar
1/2 cup granulated coconut sugar
1 tablespoon cinnamon (I used Penzey's Vietnamese Cinnamon)

Instructions:
Preheat mini-donut maker.
In a small bowl whisk together coconut flour, baking soda, cinnamon and salt.
In a medium bowl whisk together the eggs, oil and honey.
Add the dry ingredients to the wet ingredients and stir until combined.
Add the warm apple cider to the bowl and mix until fully incorporated into the dough.
Scoop the donut batter into the pre-heated donut maker. A cookie scooper makes it easy. (About 1 1/2 tablespoons for each donut)
Close the lid and cook for 2-3 minutes.
Carefully remove cooked donuts from the pan.
Either brush donuts with melted ghee/butter/coconut oil or dip them in to cover both sides.
Toss donuts with the prepared cinnamon/coconut sugar mixture until coated.

14. Prosciutto-Wrapped Mini Frittata Muffins

Ingredients:
4 tablespoons fat (coconut oil, ghee, etc.)
½ medium onion, finely diced
3 cloves of garlic, minced
½ pound of cremini mushrooms, thinly sliced
½ pound frozen spinach, thawed and squeezed dry
8 large eggs
¼ cup coconut milk (the fatty stuff at the top of the can works best)
2 tablespoons of coconut flour
1 cup of cherry tomatoes, halved
5 ounces of Prosciutto di Parma
Kosher salt
Freshly ground pepper
A regular 12 cup muffin tin
Instructions
Preheat the oven to 375°F and prepped veggies.
Heat half the coconut oil over medium heat in a large cast iron skillet and sautéed the onions until soft and translucently
Add the garlic and mushrooms and cook them until the mushroom moisture had evaporated. Then, season the filling with salt and pepper and spoon it on a plate to cool to room temperature
For the batter, Beat the eggs in a large bowl with coconut milk, coconut flour, salt, and pepper until well-mixed. Then, add the sautéed the mushrooms and spinach and stirred to combine.
Brush the remainder of the melted coconut oil onto the muffin tin and lined each cup with prosciutto, taking care to cover the bottom and sides completely.
Popp the muffins in the oven for about 20 minutes

15. Tasty Apple Almond Coconut Medley

Ingredients:
one-half apple cored and roughly diced
handful of sliced almonds
handful of unsweetened coconut
generous dose of cinnamon
1 pinch of low sodium salt
Instructions:
Pulse in the food processor to desired consistency–smaller is better for the little ones! Serve with almond milk, or creamy coconut milk.

16. Paleo Garlic Breadsticks (Just Don't Eat Them All Yourself)

Ingredients
1 1/3 cups almond flour
1/2 tsp salt
2 tbsp coconut oil, melted
3 tbsp coconut flour
1 clove garlic, minced
3 eggs, divided
1 tsp dried basil
1/2 tsp onion powder
1/2 tsp oregano
1/2 tsp baking powder
Ghee, for brushing

Instructions
Whisk two eggs together in a small bowl and set aside. In a separate bowl, add the almond flour, baking powder, salt, and coconut oil and stir. Add the beaten eggs and stir to combine.

Add the coconut flour into the bowl, one tablespoon at a time. After each tablespoon let the dough rest for a minute as the flour absorbs. Add the next tablespoon and repeat until you have dough that can be easily kneaded.

Preheat the oven to 350 degrees F. Line a baking sheet with parchment paper. Roll out the dough onto a separate piece of parchment paper. Working in small handfuls, roll the dough into a long rope. Twist the dough into your shape of choice and place on the baking sheet. Bake for 10 minutes.

Whisk the remaining egg and add a dash of water. Remove the breadsticks from the oven and brush with the egg wash, and then the minced garlic, basil, onion powder and oregano. Return to the oven and bake for 4-5 minutes more, until golden. Brush with melted ghee before serving.

Notes
Servings: 4-8 breadsticks, depending on size
Difficulty: Medium

17. Breakfast Quiche with Broccoli and Ham

Ingredients
3 tbsp of water
8 eggs
1 tsp of sea salt
1 tsp of black pepper
2 cups of broccoli chopped small
2 cups of red onions
2 cups of ham
1 tsp of coconut oil

Instructions
Bake pie dish for 5 minutes on 350 degrees fahrenheit.
Lightly steam broccoli for a couple of minutes, should turn a pretty bright green. Set aside.
Saute chopped red onions and chopped ham in coconut oil. If ham is fatty skip coconut oil, the fat will render and be enough.
Add veggies to lightly baked pie crust.
Then whisk eggs and water and add over veggies. Water helps make eggs fluffy, so does baking soda. Other recipes I googled use almond and coconut milk. Your pick.
Bake for 25-30 minutes or until desired firmness.

Notes
Tip: I always undercook food, you can always put it in the oven for longer.
Nutrition Information
Serving size: 4-6

18. Sun-Dried Tomato Quiche

INGREDIENTS
5 eggs
1 zucchini
1 onion
¼ tsp salt
¼ tsp pepper
2 tsp coconut oil
2 tomatoes, small
4 oz sundried tomatoes
¼ lb pancetta, sliced

INSTRUCTIONS
Preheat oven to 350° F.
Grease an 8-inch cast-iron skillet with 1 tsp coconut oil and set aside.
Melt 1 tsp coconut oil in a medium skillet over medium heat. Whirl the onion and zucchini in a food processor until finely shredded, then cook in the skillet until soft and translucent, about 10 minutes.
While the zucchini and onions soften, drain the oil from your sun-dried tomatoes if you're using oil-packed. Roughly chop and add to a medium mixing bowl.
Pull the pancetta slices apart with your fingers into shreds, then add to the tomatoes.
When the onions and zucchini are soft, add to the pancetta and tomatoes. Mix thoroughly and allow to cool to room temperature. Whisk in eggs, salt and pepper and pour into the cast-iron skillet.
Cook in the preheated oven for 1 hour and 15 minutes or until firm.
Serve warm.

19. Paleo Breakfast Burritos (Low-Carb)

Ingredients
For the tortillas
2 eggs
2 egg whites
1/2 cup water
4 tsp ground flaxseed
Pinch of salt
For the filling
1 avocado, diced
1/4 cup red bell pepper, finely diced
1/4 cup onion, finely diced
1/4 cup baked tilapia or other protein
Handful of spinach leaves
1 tsp coconut oil
Instructions
In a small bowl, whisk together the ingredients for the tortilla. Preheat the oven broiler.

Heat a 10-inch non-stick skillet over medium heat and coat well with coconut oil spray. Pour half of the tortilla mixture into the pan and swirl to evenly distribute. Using a metal spatula, loosen the edges of the tortilla from the pan. Cook a couple of minutes until golden brown on the bottom, and then carefully slide the spatula under the tortilla to loosen it from the bottom of the pan. Do not flip yet.

Place the pan under the broiler for 3-4 minutes until the tortilla gets a little bubbly. Remove the tortilla from the pan, setting on a piece of aluminium foil. Repeat with other half of tortilla mixture.

After the tortillas are done broiling, preheat the oven to 400 degrees F. In a separate small pan, heat the coconut oil over medium heat. Add the onions and peppers and sauté for 5-8 minutes, until soft. Add the spinach into the pan and wilt.

Place all of the fillings down the center of the tortillas and wrap tightly. Place into the oven for 5-8 minutes to set the shape of the tortilla. Enjoy!

Notes
Servings: 2
Difficulty: Medium

Paleo Diet Recipes 365 Days of Paleo and Coconut Recipes by Mercedes Del Rey

20. Bake Eggs in the Oven

Ingredients
- Eggs (however many you want)
- non-stick cooking spray (I use olive oil or coconut oil spray)
- salt and pepper, to taste

Instructions
1. Preheat oven to 350ºF and grease a muffin tin with non-stick cooking spray.
2. Crack eggs into tin. Season with salt and pepper.
3. Bake for 17 minutes or until eggs reach desired texture. All you have to do is set your oven to 350F,

21. Baked Eggs in Ham Cups

Prep Time: 5 minutes
Cook Time: 15 minutes
Ingredients:
Eggs
Ham or Turkey (I used smoked turkey)
(Optional) Scallions or what ever you like with your eggs!
Instructions
1. Preheat your oven to 400°F.
2. Grease up your Muffin/Cupcake Pan. You can either spray it down with some cooking spray, or you can do what I did which was smear some Coconut Oil all over it.
3. Fit 1 or 2 slices of ham in to each muffin cup. I used two because my ham was sliced real thin.

22. Grain-Free "French Toast" Breakfast Chalupa

Ingredients
1. 8 eggs
12 slices nitrate-free bacon
½ tsp salt
¼ tsp black pepper (or to taste)
8-10 Grain-Free Maple Cinnamon Pancakes
1½ tbsp coconut oil or butter

Instructions

Prepare pancakes and keep warm in the oven on low heat or warm setting.

Cut bacon with kitchen scissors and place in a bowl.

Heat a skillet over medium heat and add ½ tbsp coconut oil to grease the pan.

Add the bacon and stir frequently until cooked through. Drain grease and set aside.

In a large bowl, add eggs, salt & pepper and whisk until smooth & fluffy.

Heat a skillet over medium heat and add 1 tbsp coconut oil to grease the pan.

Add the egg mixture and stir as necessary to scramble the eggs.

When the eggs are about halfway firm, add the cooked bacon and continue to scramble until the eggs are firm.

Remove pancakes from warming and hold each one like a taco as you spoon the egg mixture into it dividing it evenly into each pancake.

Set 2 chalupas on each plate to serve.

Top with butter and maple syrup.

23. Paleo Sausage Balls

Ingredients
1 pound sausage
¼ cup coconut flour
2 large eggs
1 teaspoon baking soda
Instructions
Preheat oven to 350°.
Combine all ingredients. A stand mixer with the paddle attachment works well.
Form into balls 1¼ inches in diameter.
Place on a greased baking sheet and bake at 350° for 20 minutes.
Makes about 35 balls.

24. Macadamia Mix Breakfast

INGREDIENTS
1 cup raw macadamia nuts, roughly chopped
1 cup raw sunflower seeds
1 cup raw pepitas (pumpkin seeds)
1 cup coconut flakes, unsweetened
½ cup raw almonds, roughly chopped
½ cup dried apricots, roughly chopped
¼ cup ground flaxseed
1 tsp vanilla bean powder
4-6 cups coconut milk
INSTRUCTIONS
Add all ingredients except the coconut milk into a large bowl and stir until combined.
Serve individual portions and add coconut milk.
Store remaining muesli in an airtight container for several weeks.

25. Cherry Almond Muesli Recipe

INGREDIENTS
2 cups slivered almonds
1 cup chopped pecans
1 cup sunflower seeds
1 cup unsweetened shredded coconut
¼ teaspoon salt
2 tablespoons coconut oil, melted
Stevia
1 teaspoon vanilla extract
1 cup dried cherries

INSTRUCTIONS
Preheat oven to 300 degrees.
Combine nuts, seeds, coconut and salt in large bowl. Combine coconut oil, honey and vanilla in a small bowl, and then stir into nut mixture until well combined.
Bake on a rimmed cookie sheet lined with parchment paper for 18 - 20 minutes, until just lightly browned.
Add the dried cherries and toss to combine. Cool completely before serving.

26. Macadamia Mix Breakfast

INGREDIENTS
1 cup raw macadamia nuts, roughly chopped
1 cup raw sunflower seeds
1 cup raw pepitas (pumpkin seeds)
1 cup coconut flakes, unsweetened
½ cup raw almonds, roughly chopped
½ cup dried apricots, roughly chopped
¼ cup ground flaxseed
1 tsp vanilla bean powder
4-6 cups coconut milk

INSTRUCTIONS
Add all ingredients except the coconut milk into a large bowl and stir until combined.
Serve individual portions and add coconut milk.
Store remaining muesli in an airtight container for several weeks.

27. Chocco Granola Recipe

Ingredients
1 & 1/2 cup almonds
1 & 1/2 cup other nuts/seeds (or more almonds. I did a combo of pepitas, sunflower seeds and walnuts)
1 cup flax seed meal
1 cup flaked coconut (unsweetened)
Stevia to taste
1/2 tsp salt
1/3 cup Kelapo coconut oil, melted
1 egg
1/2 cup cacao nibs

Instructions
Preheat oven to 300F and line a large rimmed baking sheet with parchment paper.
In the bowl of a food processor, combine almonds and other nuts or seeds. Pulse until mixture resembles coarse crumbs with some bigger pieces in there too.
Transfer to a large bowl and add flax seed meal, flaked coconut, sweetener of choice, and salt. Drizzle with coconut oil and stir to combine.
Add egg, and toss until mixture begins to clump together. Stir in cacao nibs
Spread mixture evenly on prepared baking sheet and bake 20 minutes, stirring frequently.
Remove and let cool.

28. Cherry Almond Muesli Recipe

INGREDIENTS
2 cups slivered almonds
1 cup chopped pecans
1 cup sunflower seeds
1 cup unsweetened shredded coconut
¼ teaspoon salt
2 tablespoons coconut oil, melted
Stevia
1 teaspoon vanilla extract
1 cup dried cherries

INSTRUCTIONS
Preheat oven to 300 degrees.

Combine nuts, seeds, coconut and salt in large bowl. Combine coconut oil, honey and vanilla in a small bowl, and then stir into nut mixture until well combined.

Bake on a rimmed cookie sheet lined with parchment paper for 18 - 20 minutes, until just lightly browned.

Add the dried cherries and toss to combine. Cool completely before serving.

29. Vegetarian Curry with Squash

Ingredients:
1 tbsp coconut oil
2 cups mixed raw nuts.
1 medium yellow onion, diced
1 tsp low sodium salt
1 green bell pepper, thinly sliced
4 cloves garlic, minced
1-inch piece fresh ginger, peeled and minced
1 14-oz. can coconut milk
1 large acorn squash, peeled, seeded, and cut into 1-inch cubes
2 tsp lime juice
One teaspoon curry powder (mild or hot)
1/4 cup cilantro, chopped
Cauliflower rice, for serving

Instructions:

Melt the coconut oil in a large pan over medium heat. Add the onion and cook for 5-6 minutes, stirring occasionally. Add the bell pepper, garlic, ginger, and low sodium salt and stir to combine. Cook for an additional minute.

Add the curry powder to the pan and cook for about a minute, stirring to coat the other ingredients. Add in the coconut milk and bring to a simmer. Stir in the squash.

Simmer, stirring occasionally, for 15-20 minutes until the squash is fork-tender. Remove the pan from the heat and stir in the lime juice. Taste and adjust low sodium salt and lime juice as necessary. Sprinkle with cilantro to serve.

Roast the nuts under the grill until crisp and sprinkle over the top of the curry.

30. Spectacular Spaghetti and Delish Turkey Balls

Ingredients:
1 spaghetti squash
Extra virgin olive oil,
low sodium salt and pepper
1 tsp dried or fresh oregano
For the sauce:
1 lb ground turkey
1 small onion, chopped
4 cloves garlic, minced
1 tbsp coconut oil
1 tomato, chopped
1/2 jar of tomato sauce
1 tbsp Italian seasoning
low sodium salt and pepper to taste
Fresh basil

Instructions:
Preheat oven to 400 degrees F. Using a sharp knife, cut the squash in half lengthwise. Scoop out the seeds and discard.
Place the halves with the cut side up on a rimmed baking sheet. Drizzle with olive oil and season with low sodium salt, pepper, and oregano. Roast the squash in the oven for 40-45 minutes, until you can poke the squash easily with a fork.
Let it cool until you can handle it safely. Then scrape the insides with a fork to shred the squash into strands.
While the spaghetti squash is roasting, melt coconut oil in a large skillet over medium heat.
Add chopped onion and garlic and cook for 4-5 minutes. Add ground turkey and brown the meat, stirring occasionally. Season with low sodium salt and pepper.
Add the chopped tomato, tomato sauce, and Italian seasoning and stir to combine. Simmer on low heat, stirring occasionally, while the spaghetti squash finishes roasting. Serve over spaghetti squash with basil for garnish.

31. Sensational Courgette Pasta and Turkey Bolognaise

Ingredients:
4 medium zucchini
For the sauce:
1 lb ground turkey
1 small onion, chopped
4 cloves garlic, minced
1 tbsp coconut oil
1 tomato, chopped
1/2 jar of tomato sauce
1 tbsp Italian seasoning
low sodium salt and pepper to taste
Fresh basil, for garnish

Instructions:
Use a julienne peeler to slice the zucchini into noodles, stopping when you reach the seeds. Set aside.
If cooking zucchini noodles, simply add to a skillet and sauté over medium heat for 4-5 minutes.
Melt coconut oil in a large skillet over medium heat. Add chopped onion and garlic and cook for 4-5 minutes.
Add ground turkey and brown the meat, stirring occasionally. Season with low sodium salt and pepper.
Add the chopped tomato, tomato sauce, and Italian seasoning and stir to combine. Simmer on low heat, stirring occasionally.
Add the sauce to the noodles and ENJOY.

32. Ostrich Steak or Venison with Divine Mustard Sauce and Roasted Tomatoes

Ingredients:
For the tomatoes:
2 pints cherry tomatoes, halved
2 tbsp extra virgin olive oil
Stevia to taste
low sodium salt and freshly ground pepper
For the cauliflower rice:
1/2 head of cauliflower, chopped coarsely
1/2 small onion, finely diced
1 tbsp coconut oil
1 tbsp fresh parsley, chopped
low sodium salt and freshly ground pepper, to taste
For the meat:
4 Ostrich or venison steaks
Extra virgin olive oil
low sodium salt and freshly ground pepper
Coconut oil, for the pan
For the sauce:
1/4 cup red onion, finely diced
1/4 cup apple cider vinegar
1 cup low sodium chicken stock
1 tbsp whole grain mustard
low sodium salt and freshly ground pepper, to taste

Instructions:
Preheat the oven to 400 degrees F. Place the tomatoes on a baking sheet and drizzle with olive oil and honey. Sprinkle with low sodium salt and pepper and toss to coat evenly. Bake for 15-20 minutes until soft.

While the tomatoes are roasting, prepare the cauliflower rice. Place the cauliflower into a food processor and pulse until reduced to the size of rice grains.

Melt the coconut oil in a nonstick skillet over medium heat. Add the onion and cook for 5-6 minutes until translucent. Stir in the cauliflower, season with low sodium salt and pepper, and cover. Cook for 7-10 minutes until the cauliflower has softened, and then toss with parsley.

To make the lamb, preheat the oven to 325 degrees F. Pat the ostrich or venison dry and rub with olive oil. Generously season both sides with low sodium salt and pepper.

Heat one tablespoon of coconut oil in a cast iron skillet. When the pan is hot, add to the pan and sear for 2-3 minutes on all sides until golden brown.

Place the skillet in the oven and bake for 5-8 minutes until the ostrich or venison reaches desired doneness. Let rest for 10 minutes before serving.

While the meat is resting, add the red onion to the skillet with the pan drippings from the lamb. Sauté for 3-4 minutes, then add the white wine vinegar.

Turn the heat to high and cook until the vinegar has mostly evaporated. Add the stock and bring to a boil, cooking until the sauce reduces by half.

Stir in the mustard, and season to taste with low sodium salt and pepper. Pour over ostrich or venison to serve.

33. Tantalizing Turkey Pepper Stir-fry

Ingredients:
2 bell peppers, sliced
1 cup broccoli florets
2 cooked and shredded turkey breasts
1/4 teaspoon chili powder
low sodium salt and pepper to taste
1 tablespoon coconut oil for frying

Instructions:
Add 1 tablespoon coconut oil into a frying pan on a medium heat.
Place the sliced bell peppers into the frying pan.
After the bell peppers soften, add in the cooked turkey meat.
Add in the chili powder, low sodium salt and pepper.
Mix well and stir-fry for a few more minutes.

34. Cheeky Chicken Stir Fry

Ingredients:
1 pound boneless, skinless chicken breast
2 tablespoons coconut oil
1 medium onion, finely chopped (about 1 cup)
2 heads broccoli, sliced into 3-inch spears (about 4 cups)
2 medium carrots, sliced (about 1 cup)
2 heads baby bok choy, sliced crosswise into 1-inch strips (about 1½ cups)
4 ounces shiitake mushrooms, stemmed and thinly sliced (about 1 cup)
1 small zucchini, sliced (about 1 cup)
½ teaspoon low sodium salt
Garlic powder to taste
1½ cups water

Instructions:
Rinse the chicken and pat dry. Cut into 1-inch cubes and transfer to a plate.
Heat the coconut oil in a large skillet over medium heat
Saute the onion for 8 to 10 minutes, until soft and translucent
Add the broccoli, carrots, and chicken and saute for 10 minutes until almost tender
Add the bok choy, mushrooms, zucchini, and low sodium salt and saute for 5 minutes
Add 1 cup of the water, cover the skillet, and cook for about 10 minutes, until the vegetables are wilted
In a small bowl, dissolve the arrowroot powder in the remaining ½ cup of water, stirring until thoroughly combined
Season at the end with garlic powder, salt and if you like some chilli powder

35. Chicken Fennel Stir-Fry

Ingredients:
3 chicken breasts or the meat from 1 whole roasted chicken
2 tablespoons coconut oil
1 onion
1 bulb of fennel
1 teaspoon each of low sodium salt, pepper, garlic powder and basil
Instructions:
Stovetop:
Cut the chicken into bite sized pieces. If chicken is raw, heat butter/coconut oil in large skillet or wok until melted.
Add chicken and cook on medium/high heat until chicken is cooked through. (If chicken is pre-cooked, cook the vegetables first then add chicken)
While cooking, cut the onion into bite sized pieces (1/2 inch) and thinly slice the fennel bulb into thin slivers.
Add all to skillet or wok, add spices and continue sautéing until all are cooked through and fragrant.
This will take approximately 10-12 minutes.

36. Muddy Buddy Recipe

INGREDIENTS
Cereal:
2 Cups almond flour
½ Cup + 2 tablespoons arrowroot starch/flour
2 Tablespoons ground flax seed
1 Teaspoon baking soda
Pinch of salt
⅓ Cup melted coconut oil
1 Teaspoon pure vanilla extract
3 Tablespoons unsweetened almond milk
Stevia to taste
Muddy Buddies:
¼ Cup sunbutter (or nut butter of choice)
⅓ Cup Enjoy Life Chocolate Chips
1 Tablespoons coconut oil
⅓-1/2 Cup powdered coconut sugar
Powdered Coconut Sugar:
1 Cup coconut sugar
1 Tablespoons arrowroot starch

INSTRUCTIONS
Preheat oven to 350 degrees.
In a large mixing bowl, combine the flour, flaxseed, arrowroot, baking soda and salt. Mix in the remaining cereal ingredients, and combine until a dough forms.
Line 2 baking sheets with parchment paper.
Lay the dough on a separate large sheet of parchment paper, and roll out into a thin square. You want the dough to be about ¼ inch thick. Use a pizza or pastry cutter to cut the dough into small squares.
Using a small spatula (I used a pie server) transfer the small squares to the baking sheets. Lay them close together, but make sure they aren't touching. Separating the squares takes the most time, but is very easy. This is a great place to have little hands help out.
Place both baking sheets in the oven and cook for 4 minutes, or until the undersides of the cereal pieces are beginning to lightly brown. Flip the cereal pieces and rotate the baking sheets (optional but will ensure even baking). Return to the oven for 4-5 minutes or until browned and cooked through. Baking time will vary by the size of your cereal pieces so keep an eye on the cereal while it cooks. Set aside the cereal to cool completely.
Now begin the muddy buddies.
Make the powdered coconut sugar by blending the coconut sugar and arrowroot in a high speed blender on high until powdered. Make sure the lid is on tight, or you'll have powdered coconut sugar everywhere!
In a small saucepan over medium-low heat, combine the sunbutter, chocolate chips and coconut oil until smooth. Let cool for a minute.
Place the cooled cereal in a large mixing bowl and pour the chocolate mixture on top. Stir so that it is all well coated.
Place the coated cereal in a ziplock baggie, pour the ⅓-1/2 cup of powdered coconut sugar on top and toss until the cereal is coated in powdered sugar.
Place in a serving bowl and sprinkle with more coconut sugar to taste.

NOTES
Store the muddy buddies at room temperature in a closed container.
The cereal can be made a day in advance and stored at room temperature in a sealed baggie or container.

37. Creamy Chicken Casserole

Ingredients:
2 cups cubed cooked chicken
1 1/2 cups cooked butternut squash
1/2 cup coconut cream,
1/4 cup coconut oil, melted
1 heaping cup green peas, fresh or frozen
1 tbsp apple cider vinegar
1/2 tsp low sodium salt
1/2 tsp oregano
1/2 tsp thyme
1 tbsp fresh parsley

Instructions:
In a large bowl, mash the butternut squash. Stir in the coconut cream, oil, vinegar, low sodium salt, oregano, and thyme. Once everything is combined, add in chicken and peas.
Place the mixture into a large saucepan and cook over medium heat for 5-8 minutes.
Top with fresh parsley and serve warm.

38. Vegetarian Curry with Squash

Ingredients:
1 tbsp coconut oil
2 cups mixed raw nuts.
1 medium yellow onion, diced
1 tsp low sodium salt
1 green bell pepper, thinly sliced
4 cloves garlic, minced
1-inch piece fresh ginger, peeled and minced
1 14-oz. can coconut milk
1 large acorn squash, peeled, seeded, and cut into 1-inch cubes
2 tsp lime juice
One teaspoon curry powder (mild or hot)
1/4 cup cilantro, chopped
Cauliflower rice, for serving

Instructions:

Melt the coconut oil in a large pan over medium heat. Add the onion and cook for 5-6 minutes, stirring occasionally. Add the bell pepper, garlic, ginger, and low sodium salt and stir to combine. Cook for an additional minute.

Add the curry powder to the pan and cook for about a minute, stirring to coat the other ingredients. Add in the coconut milk and bring to a simmer. Stir in the squash.

Simmer, stirring occasionally, for 15-20 minutes until the squash is fork-tender. Remove the pan from the heat and stir in the lime juice. Taste and adjust low sodium salt and lime juice as necessary. Sprinkle with cilantro to serve.

Roast the nuts under the grill until crisp and sprinkle over the top of the curry.

39. Red Cabbage Bonanza Salad

Ingredients:
For the chicken or turkey:
450g chicken/turkey mince, free range of course
1 long red chili, finely chopped with the seeds
2 garlic cloves, finely chopped
Little nob of fresh ginger, peeled and finely chopped
1 stem lemon grass, pale section only, finely chopped
1/2 bunch of coriander stems washed and finely chopped (I don't waste anything, save the leaves for the salad)
1 tbsp low sodium salt
1 tbsp coconut aminos
1/2 lime rind grated
1/2 lime, juiced
A pinch of low sodium salt
Coconut oil for frying (about 3 tablespoons)
For the salad:
1/4 red cabbage, thinly sliced
1 large carrot, peeled and grated
1/2 Spanish onion, thinly sliced
2 tbsps green spring onion, chopped
1/2 bunch of fresh coriander leaves (saved from the stems used in the chicken)
A handful of fresh mint or Thai basil if available
1/2 cup crashed roasted cashews or some sesame seeds
1/2 cup dried fried shallots (optional for garnish)
2 tbsp toasted coconut flakes (optional for garnish)
For the dressing:
2 tbsp olive oil
3 tbsps lime juice
1 small red chili, finely chopped (you can leave it out if you like it mild)
Instructions:
Once you've prepared all your ingredients for the chicken, heat 1 tbsp of coconut oil in a large frying pan or a wok to high. Throw in lemongrass, chili, garlic, coriander stems and ginger and stir fry for about a minute until fragrant.
Add chicken mince and lime zest. Stir and break apart the mince with a wooden mixing spoon until separated into small
The meat will now be changing to white colour. Add lime juice. Stir through and cook for a further few minutes. Total cooking time for the chicken should be about 10 minutes.
Prepare the salad base by mixing together sliced red cabbage, onion grated carrot, and fresh herbs.
Mix all dressing ingredients and toss through the salad.
Serve cooked chicken mince on top of the dressed salad and topped with roasted cashews, dried shallots, coconut flakes and extra fresh herbs.

40. Paleo Crock Pot Cashew Chicken

Ingredients
1. 1/4 cup arrowroot starch
2. 1/2 tsp. black pepper
3. 2 lbs. chicken thighs, cut into bite-size pieces
4. 1 tbs. coconut oil
5. 3 tbs. coconut aminos
6. 2 tbs. rice wine vinegar
7. 2 tbs. organic ketchup (tomato paste would work also)
8. 1/2-1 tbs. palm sugar
9. 2 minced garlic cloves
10. 1/2 tsp. minced fresh ginger
11. 1/4-1/2 red pepper flakes
12. 1/2 cup raw cashews

Instructions
1. Place starch and black pepper in a large Ziploc bag. Add chicken pieces and seal; toss to thoroughly coat meat.
2. Melt coconut oil in a large skillet or wok. Add chicken and cook for about 5 minutes until brown on all sides. Remove and add to crock pot.
3. Mix coconut aminos through red pepper flakes in a small bowl. Pour mixture over chicken and toss to coat. Put lid on crock pot and cook on low for 3-4 hours.
4. Stir cashews into chicken and sauce before serving.

41. Spicy Slow Cooker Chorizo Chili

Ingredients
1 pound of grass fed beef
2 fresh chorizo sausages, casings removed (about 1/2 pound)
1 onion, diced
1 teaspoon of minced garlic
1 15 oz can of tomato sauce
1 15 oz can of diced tomatoes
1 can of rotel, I used hot
2 chipotle peppers in adobo, chopped
2 Tablespoons of chili powder
1 Tablespoon of cumin
salt and pepper to taste

Instructions
brown off all the meat in a skillet
drain and toss in the crock pot
in the same skillet add onions and garlic and cook just long enough to get some colour on those onions (you may skip this step and just toss it in the crock pot, but I just personally like to get some colour on the onions before adding them in)
toss remaining ingredients in the crock pot and stir together
cook on low for 6-8 hours or on high for 4-6 hours
top with diced avocado, minced red onion and cilantro to serve

42. Crock-Pot Roast

Ingredients
4 lb (1816g) beef chuck roast
1 tbsp (14g) light oil (for sautéing ... such as coconut, olive or ghee)
1 cup (232g) red wine, good quality
4 each (12g) garlic cloves
10 sprigs (10g) fresh thyme
1 each (.64g) bay leaf
1 large (72g) carrot, peeled and cut into chunks
2 each (101g) celery ribs, cut into chunks
1 small (110g) onion, cut into chunks
1 small (420g) head cauliflower, leaves removed and cut into florets
salt and fresh cracked pepper, to taste

Instructions:
1. Turn on your slow cooker, setting it to low.
2. Season your beef with a good layer and salt and pepper.
3. Heat a large sauté pan or skillet over medium high heat. Add your oil to the pan and swirl it around. Quickly add your beef to the pan and sear it, until a nice brown crust has formed. Flip it over and sear the other side. Continue flipping it, until all sides have been properly seared. Add your beef to the crock pot.
4. Pour your red wine into the still very hot pan, with all the "stuff" stuck to the bottom. This should QUICKLY boil, releasing some of those little flavour morsels into the hot wine. Swirl the pan around and use a wooden spoon to scrape anything else off the bottom of the pan, into the wine. Pour the wine mixture over the top of the beef.
5. Add your garlic, thyme and bay leaves to the slow cooker, making sure it's pushed into the liquid.
6. Add the rest of the vegetables, except the cauliflower. Season with a bit of salt and pepper. Again, push these into the areas on the side of the roast, as much as possible. You don't want much of it covering the roast. You want most of the veggies on the sides, surrounding the roast. As this all cooks, the meat and veggies will shrink, releasing their juices, creating an AMAZING flavour, as well as creating its own natural juices, in which to cook! Getting everything as close to the bottom of the pot, as is possible, will help this process along.
7. Add the lid and allow the ingredients to cook for 8 hours.
8. After 8 hours, add your cauliflower to the pot and push the florets under the surface of the liquid, as much as possible. Season with a bit of salt and pepper. Cover and allow to cook for 20 minutes.
9. Serve!

43. Paleo Mini Meatloaves

Ingredients
2 pounds ground meat – mixture of grass fed beef and/or pork and/or veal
10 ounces frozen, chopped spinach
1-2 teaspoons oil
1 medium onion, finely diced
6 ounces mushrooms, finely diced
2 carrots, grated or finely diced
4 eggs, lightly beaten
1/3 cup coconut flour
2 teaspoons salt
2 teaspoons pepper
2 teaspoons onion powder
1 teaspoon garlic powder
1 teaspoon dried thyme
1/4 teaspoon grated nutmeg

Instructions
Preheat oven to 375 degrees F
Thaw the spinach, squeeze out the excess water and set aside.
Heat a pan on medium heat, add the oil and fry the onions and mushrooms until the onions are translucent and some of the liquid has cooked out of the mushrooms. Set aside to cool.
Place the ground meat in a large bowl, add the spinach, carrots, mushroom/onion mixture, beaten eggs, coconut flour and all the spices. Use your hands to combine it well but do not overmix.
Fill 18 regular size muffin tins to the top with the meatloaf mixture. (Greasing the tins may be a good idea if the meat you're using is fairly lean)
Cook for 20-25 minutes or until internal temperature reaches 160 degrees.
Allow to cool and use a knife to loosen meatloaves from sides of the pan before removing.

44. Kale and Red Pepper Frittata

Ingredients
1 tbsp coconut oil
1/2 cup chopped red pepper
1/3 cup chopped onion
3 slices crispy bacon, chopped
2 cups chopped kale, de-stemmed and rinsed
8 large eggs
1/2 cup almond or coconut milk
Salt and pepper to taste

Instructions
Preheat oven to 350 degrees. In a medium bowl, whisk the eggs and milk together. Add salt and pepper. Set aside.
In a non-stick skillet, heat about a tablespoon of coconut oil over medium heat. Add onion and red pepper and sauté for 3 minutes, until onion is translucent. Add kale and cook until it wilts, about 5 minutes.
Add eggs to the pan mixture, along with the bacon. Cook for about 4 minutes until the bottom and edges of the frittata start to set.
Put frittata in the oven and cook for 10-15 minutes until the frittata is cooked all the way through. Slice and serve.

Notes
Servings: 4
Difficulty: Easy

45. The Best Homemade Ranch Dressing Ever

Ingredients
1/2 cup Paleo mayo (see below)
1/2 cup coconut milk
1/2 tsp onion powder
1 tsp garlic powder
1 tsp dill
Salt and freshly ground pepper, to taste

Instructions
Whisk all ingredients together to combine. Season with salt and pepper to taste. Store in an airtight container in the refrigerator for up to a week.

Mayo recipe
1 egg, room temperature
2 tbsp lemon juice or apple cider vinegar
1/2 tsp salt
1/2 tsp dry mustard
1 cup light olive oil*

In a tall glass (if using an immersion blender) or a blender, place the egg and lemon juice. Let come to room temperature, about one hour. Add the salt and mustard. Blend ingredients. While blending, very slowly pour in the olive oil. Blend until it reaches desired consistency. Store in the refrigerator for up to a week.

*It's important to use a light olive oil, not full flavour, for mayonnaise. You could also use almond or walnut oil instead.

46. Skinny Eggie Vegetable Stir Fry

Ingredients:
1 lb of Cubed Butternut Squash
1 lb of Green Beans
3 Baby Bok Choys
1½ lb of Eggplants
3 Garlic Cloves
1 small Yellow Onion
½ teaspoon of low sodium salt
½ teaspoon of Black Pepper
1-2 Tablespoons of coconut oil
3 organic eggs

Instructions:
Peel, core, and cut the butternut squash into 1" cubes.
Snap the ends off the green beans and slice at an angle into 1.5" long pieces.
Chop the bok choy leaves from the stems. Slice the stems into 1" thick pieces. Cut the leaves in half.
Slice the eggplants into 1" thick discs, then quarter the disc into wedges. Slice in half if the eggplant is skinny.
Mince the garlic cloves and slice the onions.
Heat a wok and add the cooking oil.
Add the onions and cook until translucent. About 2 minutes.
Add the garlic and cook for another minute.
Add the squash, beans (see note), low sodium salt, pepper
Add the eggplant and bok choy stalks and cook uncovered for another 7-10 minutes.
Add the bok choy leaves and cook for another few minutes, covered.
Beat the eggs and add them to the stir fry …keep stirring till they are cooked through

47. Easy Paleo Slow Cooker Pot Roast

Ingredients
3 lbs. boneless beef roast, trimmed of fat
1 tbsp coconut oil
1 cup beef stock
5 carrots, peeled and diced
2 stalks celery, diced
1/2 large onion, sliced
3 garlic cloves, chopped
1 tbsp fresh parsley, chopped
For the spice rub
1 tbsp freshly ground black pepper
1 tbsp ground coriander
2 tsp cinnamon
1 1/2 tsp salt
1/2 tsp ground clove
1/2 tsp ground allspice
Instructions
Mix together the ingredients for the spice rub and massage into the roast. Heat the coconut oil in a large skillet over medium-high heat. Add the roast to the pan and let sear for 5 minutes. Flip and repeat with the other side. Transfer the roast to the slow cooker.

Add the carrots, onion, garlic, and celery to the slow cooker. Pour in the broth. Turn the heat on to low and cook for 6-7 hours, until the meat is tender. Serve hot sprinkled with chopped parsley.
Notes
Servings: 6
Difficulty: Easy

48. Red Cabbage Bonanza Salad

Ingredients:
For the chicken or turkey:
450g chicken/turkey mince, free range of course
1 long red chili, finely chopped with the seeds
2 garlic cloves, finely chopped
Little nob of fresh ginger, peeled and finely chopped
1 stem lemon grass, pale section only, finely chopped
1/2 bunch of coriander stems washed and finely chopped (I don't waste anything, save the leaves for the salad)
1 tbsp low sodium salt
1 tbsp coconut aminos
1/2 lime rind grated
1/2 lime, juiced
A pinch of low sodium salt
Coconut oil for frying (about 3 tablespoons)
For the salad:
1/4 red cabbage, thinly sliced
1 large carrot, peeled and grated
1/2 Spanish onion, thinly sliced
2 tbsps green spring onion, chopped
1/2 bunch of fresh coriander leaves (saved from the stems used in the chicken)
A handful of fresh mint or Thai basil if available
1/2 cup crashed roasted cashews or some sesame seeds
1/2 cup dried fried shallots (optional for garnish)
2 tbsp toasted coconut flakes (optional for garnish)
For the dressing:
2 tbsp olive oil
3 tbsps lime juice
1 small red chili, finely chopped (you can leave it out if you like it mild)
Instructions:
Once you've prepared all your ingredients for the chicken, heat 1 tbsp of coconut oil in a large frying pan or a wok to high. Throw in lemongrass, chili, garlic, coriander stems and ginger and stir fry for about a minute until fragrant.
Add chicken mince and lime zest. Stir and break apart the mince with a wooden mixing spoon until separated into small
The meat will now be changing to white colour. Add lime juice. Stir through and cook for a further few minutes. Total cooking time for the chicken should be about 10 minutes.
Prepare the salad base by mixing together sliced red cabbage, onion grated carrot, and fresh herbs.
Mix all dressing ingredients and toss through the salad.
Serve cooked chicken mince on top of the dressed salad and topped with roasted cashews, dried shallots, coconut flakes and extra fresh herbs.

49. Sausage and Kale "Pasta" Casserole

Ingredients
1 lb. Italian sausage
1 medium spaghetti squash, halved and seeded
Extra virgin olive oil, for drizzling
1 large bunch of kale, de-stemmed, and chopped
1/2 red onion, sliced thin
1/3 cup chicken broth
1/2 cup coconut milk
1 clove garlic, minced
2 tsp Italian seasoning
Salt and freshly ground pepper, to taste

Instructions
Preheat the oven to 400 degrees F. Place the squash in the microwave for 3-4 minutes to soften. Using a sharp knife, cut the squash in half lengthwise. Scoop out the seeds and discard. Place the halves, with the cut side up, on a rimmed baking sheet. Drizzle with olive oil and sprinkle with salt and pepper. Roast in the oven for 45-50 minutes, until you can poke the squash easily with a fork. Let it cool until you can handle it safely. Then scrape the insides with a fork to shred the squash into strands.

Meanwhile, melt the coconut oil in a large oven-safe skillet over medium heat. Add the sausage and brown. Once cooked through, remove to a plate. In the same skillet, add the onion and sauté for 3-4 minutes. Next add the garlic, Italian seasoning, and kale and cook for 2-3 minutes to slightly wilt the kale. Pour in the chicken broth and coconut milk and simmer for an additional 2-3 minutes. Remove from heat.

Stir in the cooked sausage. Add the spaghetti squash into the skillet and stir well to combine. Bake for 15-18 minutes, until the top has slightly browned. Serve hot.

Notes
Servings: 4
Difficulty: Medium

50. Divine Chicken or Turkey and Baby Bok Choy Salad

Ingredients:
For the salad:
2 cups grilled chicken or turkey, chopped
6 baby bok choy, grilled & chopped
2 green onions, chopped
1/4 cup cilantro, chopped
1 Tbsp sesame seeds
For the dressing:
1 Tbsp fresh ginger, chopped
2 Tbsp coconut cream
1 Tbsp soy sauce
1 Tbsp sesame oil
2 Tbsp fresh lime juice
1 Tsp stevia powder
Instructions:
Combine all of the salad ingredients until well mixed.
Add all of the ingredients for the dressing into a blender or food processor, and blend until mostly smooth
Pour the dressing over the salad and toss lightly until coated.
Garnish with more sesame seeds if desired.

51. Broiled Curry Coconut Sole or Cod

Ingredients:
1 tsp dark sesame oil, divided
1 tbsp minced peeled fresh ginger
4 garlic cloves, minced
1 cup finely chopped red bell pepper
1 cup chopped scallions
1 tsp curry powder
2 tsp red curry paste
1/2 tsp ground cumin
4 tsp low-sodium soy sauce
Stevia to taste
1 (14-ounce) can light coconut milk
1/4 cup chopped fresh cilantro
6 (6-ounce) fish fillets
Low sodium salt
Cooking spray

Instructions:
Preheat broiler.
Heat 1/2 teaspoon oil in a large nonstick skillet over medium heat. Add ginger and garlic; cook 1 minute. Add pepper and scallions; cook 1 minute. Stir in curry powder, curry paste, and cumin; cook 1 minute. Add soy sauce, stevia, and coconut milk; bring to a simmer (do not boil). Remove from heat; stir in cilantro or basil if using.
Brush fish with 1/2 teaspoon oil; sprinkle with 1/4 teaspoon low sodium salt. Place fish on a baking sheet coated with cooking spray. Broil 7 minutes or until fish flakes easily when tested with a fork. Serve fish with sauce and lime wedges.
Serve with cauliflower rice

52. Sexy Shrimp on Sticks

Ingredients:
1/2 lb shrimp, peeled and deveined
1/4 cup coconut milk
1 tsp fish sauce
6 gloves garlic, chopped
1/4 tsp each turmeric, cumin, low sodium salt

Instructions:

Heat olive oil in a large pan over medium heat. Add onion and garlic and cook until tender. Add chili flake and stir for about a minute.

When that has cooked down, add the diced tomatoes and oregano. Simmer for about 10 minutes.

Add julienned zucchini and lemon juice and cook, stirring, for about 5 minutes.

Add shrimp and then the spinach, once shrimp is just cooked through. Low sodium salt and pepper to taste and serve with a fresh squeeze of lemon.

53. Delicious Fish Stir Fry

Ingredients:
200 grams any white fish fillet (cut into pieces)
1 Tablespoon Coconut Vinegar
1/2 Teaspoon Ginger and Garlic fresh pressed
1 small onion (quartered)
1/2 Cup Bell Peppers de-seeded and cubed (Red or Yellow).
1/2 Cup Mushrooms (any kind)
2 to 3 stalks of scallions (cut into 1.5 inch length)
low sodium salt to taste
1 Teaspoon Chili powder (Optional)
1 Teaspoon Fish Sauce
1/2 Tablespoon Extra Virgin Olive Oil

Instructions:
Put a pot with a bit of low sodium salt to boil and make sure your rice noodles are handy. Later, when the water has boiled, pop the noodles in and give it a stir.
Heat 2 tbsp. coconut oil in a wok or large pan.
Add the sliced garlic and grated ginger to the wok and stir-fry for 30 seconds.
Add the green onion and stir-fry 1 more minute.
Add the carrot and stir-fry about a minute. You want it just barely cooked, not limp and soggy. Remove the vegetable mixture to a bowl and set aside.
Add another 2/3 tbsp. of coconut oil to the wok.
When the oil is very hot, add the green pepper and stir-fry for 1 minute.
Heat a ½ tbsp. of coconut oil, then add the pieces of turkey breast and stir-fry. I found that the turkey got some color from the previous ingredients that were in the wok. If this doesn't happen, add a tiny amount of soy sauce.
Stir-fry until just done and no more. To check, I like to cut open the biggest piece to make sure it isn't pink in the middle.
Add the sesame oil.

54. Spectacular Salmon

Ingredients:
For the salmon:
2 salmon fillets (6oz each)
1 heaping tablespoon coconut flour
2 tablespoons fresh parsley
1 tablespoon olive oil
1 tablespoon mustard powder
low sodium salt and pepper, to taste
For the salad:
2 cups any green leaf salad
¼ red onion, sliced thin
juice of 1 lemon
1 tablespoon white wine vinegar
1 tablespoon olive oil
low sodium salt and pepper, to taste
Instructions:
Preheat oven to 375F.

Mix the chopped raw shrimp, egg, onions, parsley, almond meal, 1tbsp coconut butter, garlic, low sodium salt and pepper. Set aside.

Lightly season the salmon pieces with low sodium salt and pepper. Heat a cast iron pan on high and add the rest of the lard. Pan sear the salmon 1-2 minutes per side.

Move the salmon to an ovenproof dish and top each piece with 2 tbsp (or more!) of the shrimp topping. Lightly brush the top with a little bit of lard and bake in the oven for 15 minutes.

Afterwards, set your oven to broil and cook for about 3 more minutes until the top becomes crispy.

55. Creamy Coconut Salmon

Ingredients:
1 pound wild salmon fillets
¼ tsp low sodium salt
¼ tsp freshly ground black pepper
2 tsp coconut oil
3 cloves fresh garlic (minced)
1 large shallot (minced)
1 lemon (juice and zest)
½ cup unsweetened full-fat coconut milk

Instructions:
Preheat oven to 450 degrees.
Place salmon fillets on a parchment or foil lined baking sheet.
Top your salmon off with olive oil and mustard powder and rub into your salmon.
In a small bowl, mix together your coconut flour, parsley, and low sodium salt and pepper.
Use a spoon to sprinkle on your toppings on your salmon and then your hand to pat into your salmon.
Place in oven for 10-15 minutes or until salmon is cooked to your preference. I cooked mine more on the medium rare side at 12 minutes.
While the salmon is cooking, mix together your salad ingredients.
When salmon is done, place salmon on top of salad and consume.

56. Salmon Dill Bonanza

Ingredients:
1 1/2 pounds wild salmon (I used sockeye)
zest of one lemon (about a tablespoon)
2 tablespoons oil
1 tablespoon chopped, fresh dill
1 lemon
low sodium salt and pepper

Instructions:
Preheat oven to 375°F.
Place salmon in a shallow baking dish and season with low sodium salt and pepper.
Heat coconut oil in a medium saute pan or cast iron skillet over medium heat. Add garlic and shallots and saute until tender and fragrant, 3-5 minutes.
Add lemon zest, lemon juice, and coconut milk, stirring to combine.
Bring to a low boil, then remove from heat.
Pour mixture over salmon. Bake, uncovered, for 10-20 minutes or until salmon flakes easily with a fork.

57. Sexy Shrimp Cocktail

Ingredients:
1 pound uncooked shrimp, peeled, deveined, and thawed if frozen
1 tablespoon olive oil
Low sodium salt and fresh ground pepper to taste
1 cup coconut cream and two tablespoon tomato paste
One teaspoon fresh pressed garlic
lemon wedges

Instructions:
Preheat oven to 400 degrees F.
Oil the bottom of a 9 x 13 baking dish.
Rinse the salmon and pat dry with paper towels. Sprinkle with low sodium salt and pepper and place in the prepared dish.
Mix together the oil (room temperature), lemon zest and dill.
Place about half the mixture on top of the seasoned salmon. You can spread the lemon dill mixture or leave it in dollops like this.
Bake for about 10-15 minutes. The salmon will continue cooking even after you take it out of the oven.
Add the remaining oil/dill/lemon zest mixture on top, add a squeeze of lemon juice.

58. Gambas al Ajillo--Sizzling Garlic Shrimp

Ingredients:
1/2 cup olive oil
10 cloves garlic, peeled and thinly sliced
1 pound raw shrimp, peeled, deveined, and tails removed, defrosted if frozen
Low sodium salt and pepper to taste
1/4 teaspoon paprika
Pinch or two of red pepper flakes, optional

Instructions:
Preheat oven to 425 degrees.
Toss shrimp with oil, low sodium salt and pepper and spread in single layer on rimmed baking sheet.
Roast, turning once, until shrimp is pink and just cooked through (about 5-10 minutes, depending on size of shrimp).
Serve chilled with the blend of coconut cream, tomato paste and pressed garlic...add black pepper and lemon wedges.

59. Spicy Granola

Ingredients:
1 ½ cups almond flour
1/3 cup coconut oil
2 tsp cinnamon
2 tsp nutmeg
2 tsp vanilla extract
½ cup walnuts
½ cup coconut flakes
¼ cup hemp seeds
low sodium salt, to taste

Instructions:
Preheat oven to 275 degrees Fahrenheit.
Combine all ingredients in a large mixing bowl and mix well. (I find it easier to melt down the coconut oil a little bit before adding it)
Spread mixture into one flat layer on a greased baking sheet.
Bake for 40-50 minutes, or until mixture is toasted to your liking.
Remove from oven and allow to cool before serving, then transfer into a plastic container to save the rest!

60. Scrambled Eggs with Chilli

Ingredients:
4 fresh green chillies with skins removed
2 tablespoons (30g or 1 oz) coconut oil
1 small onion, peeled and finely chopped
6 eggs
1/4 cup (62ml or 2 fl oz) coconut milk
1/4 teaspoon (1ml) low sodium salt

Instructions:
After removing chilli skins, remove and discard seeds and finely chop remaining chilli.
Beat eggs, coconut milk and salt in a bowl and set aside.
Heat oil in a medium size saucepan over a medium heat.
Reduce heat to low and add egg mixture to saucepan and mix well.
Scatter chillies over mixture.
Cook over a low heat until eggs are cooked.
Serves 4. Serve hot.

61. Spicy India Omelet

Ingredients:
3 Eggs
1 Onion, chopped
4 Green Chilli (optional)
1/4 cup Coconut grated
Low sodium Salt, Oil - as required

Instructions:
Beat the Eggs severely.
Mix chopped onion, rounded green chilli, salt and grated coconuts with eggs.
Heat oil on a medium-low heat, in a pan.
Pour the mixture in the form of pancakes and cook it on the both sides.

62. Mushrooms, Eggs and Onion Bonanza

Ingredients:
1 medium onion, finely diced
1/4 cup coconut oil
10-12 medium white mushrooms, finely chopped
12 hard boiled eggs, peeled and finely chopped
Freshly ground black pepper to taste

Instructions:
Saute the onion in coconut oil until golden brown.
Add the mushrooms and saute another 5 minutes or so, stirring frequently, until mushrooms are softened and turned dark.
Remove from heat and let cool.
Mix together with the eggs and pepper. Chill until ready to serve.

63. Spicy Turkey Stir Fry

Ingredients:
2 lbs. boneless skinless chicken or turkey breasts, cut into 1-inch slices
2 tbsp coconut oil
1 tsp cumin seeds
1/2 each green, red, and orange bell pepper, thinly sliced
1 tsp garam masala
2 tsp freshly ground pepper
low sodium salt, to taste
Scallions, for garnish
For the marinade:
1/2 cup coconut cream
1 clove garlic, minced
1 tsp ginger, minced
1 tbsp freshly ground pepper
2 tsp low sodium salt
1/4 tsp turmeric

Instructions:
Place all of the marinade ingredients into a Ziploc bag. Add the chicken, close the bag, and shake to coat.
Marinate in the refrigerator for at least 30 minutes, or up to 6 hours.
In a wok or large sauté pan, melt the coconut oil over medium-high heat. Add the cumin seeds and cook for 2-3 minutes.
Add the marinated chicken and let cook for 5 minutes. Stir the chicken until it begins to brown, and then add the peppers, garam masala, and freshly ground pepper.
Sprinkle with low sodium salt. Cook for 4-5 minutes, stirring regularly, or until the bell pepper is cooked to desired doneness. Serve hot.

64. Turkey and Kale Pasta Casserole

Ingredients:
1 lb. Turkey breast
1 medium spaghetti squash, halved and seeded
Extra virgin olive oil, for drizzling
1 large bunch of kale, de-stemmed, and chopped
1/2 red onion, sliced thin
1/3 cup chicken broth
1/2 cup coconut milk
1 clove garlic, minced
2 tsp Italian seasoning
low sodium salt and freshly ground pepper, to taste

Instructions:
Preheat the oven to 400 degrees F. Place the squash in the microwave for 3-4 minutes to soften.
Using a sharp knife, cut the squash in half lengthwise. Scoop out the seeds and discard. Place the halves, with the cut side up, on a rimmed baking sheet.
Drizzle with olive oil and sprinkle with low sodium salt and pepper. Roast in the oven for 45-50 minutes, until you can poke the squash easily with a fork.
Let it cool until you can handle it safely. Then scrape the insides with a fork to shred the squash into strands.
Meanwhile, melt the coconut oil in a large oven-safe skillet over medium heat.
Add the turkey breast and brown. Once cooked through, remove to a plate. In the same skillet, add the onion and sauté for 3-4 minutes.
Next add the garlic, Italian seasoning, and kale and cook for 2-3 minutes to slightly wilt the kale.
Pour in the chicken broth and coconut milk and simmer for an additional 2-3 minutes. Remove from heat.
Stir in the cooked turkey. Add the spaghetti squash into the skillet and stir well to combine.
Bake for 15-18 minutes, until the top has slightly browned. Serve hot.

65. Roasted and Filled Tasty Bell Peppers

Ingredients:
5 large bell peppers
1 tbsp coconut oil
1/2 large onion, diced
1 tsp dried oregano
1/2 tsp low sodium salt
1 lb. ground turkey
1 large zucchini, halved and diced
3 tbsp tomato paste
Freshly ground black pepper, to taste
Fresh parsley, for serving

Instructions:
Preheat the oven to 350 degrees F. Coat a small baking dish with coconut oil spray. Bring a large pot of water to a boil. Cut the stems and very top of the peppers off, removing the seeds. Place in boiling water for 4-5 minutes. Remove from the water and drain face-down on a paper towel.

Heat the coconut oil in a large nonstick pan over medium heat. Add in the onion. Sauté for 3-4 minutes until the onion begins to soften. Stir in the ground turkey, oregano, low sodium salt, and pepper and cook until turkey is browned.

Add the zucchini to the skillet as the turkey finishes cooking. Cook everything together until the zucchini is soft, and then drain any juices from the pan.

Remove the pan from heat and stir in the tomato paste. Bake for 15 minutes.

66. Creamy Chicken Casserole

Ingredients:
2 cups cubed cooked chicken
1 1/2 cups cooked butternut squash
1/2 cup coconut cream,
1/4 cup coconut oil, melted
1 heaping cup green peas, fresh or frozen
1 tbsp apple cider vinegar
1/2 tsp low sodium salt
1/2 tsp oregano
1/2 tsp thyme
1 tbsp fresh parsley

Instructions:
In a large bowl, mash the butternut squash. Stir in the coconut cream, oil, vinegar, low sodium salt, oregano, and thyme.
Once everything is combined, add in chicken and peas.
Place the mixture into a large saucepan and cook over medium heat for 5-8 minutes.
Top with fresh parsley and serve warm.

67. Spectacular Spaghetti and Delish Turkey Balls

Ingredients:
1 spaghetti squash
Extra virgin olive oil,
low sodium salt and pepper
1 tsp dried or fresh oregano
For the sauce:
1 lb ground turkey
1 small onion, chopped
4 cloves garlic, minced
1 tbsp coconut oil
1 tomato, chopped
1/2 jar of tomato sauce
1 tbsp Italian seasoning
low sodium salt and pepper to taste
Fresh basil

Instructions:
Preheat oven to 400 degrees F. Using a sharp knife, cut the squash in half lengthwise. Scoop out the seeds and discard.
Place the halves with the cut side up on a rimmed baking sheet. Drizzle with olive oil and season with low sodium salt, pepper, and oregano. Roast the squash in the oven for 40-45 minutes, until you can poke the squash easily with a fork.
Let it cool until you can handle it safely. Then scrape the insides with a fork to shred the squash into strands.
While the spaghetti squash is roasting, melt coconut oil in a large skillet over medium heat.
Add chopped onion and garlic and cook for 4-5 minutes. Add ground turkey and brown the meat, stirring occasionally. Season with low sodium salt and pepper.
Add the chopped tomato, tomato sauce, and Italian seasoning and stir to combine. Simmer on low heat, stirring occasionally, while the spaghetti squash finishes roasting. Serve over spaghetti squash with basil for garnish.

68. Sensational Courgette Pasta and Turkey Bolognaise

Ingredients:
4 medium zucchini
For the sauce:
1 lb ground turkey
1 small onion, chopped
4 cloves garlic, minced
1 tbsp coconut oil
1 tomato, chopped
1/2 jar of tomato sauce
1 tbsp Italian seasoning
low sodium salt and pepper to taste
Fresh basil, for garnish

Instructions:
Use a julienne peeler to slice the zucchini into noodles, stopping when you reach the seeds. Set aside.
If cooking zucchini noodles, simply add to a skillet and sauté over medium heat for 4-5 minutes.
Melt coconut oil in a large skillet over medium heat. Add chopped onion and garlic and cook for 4-5 minutes.
Add ground turkey and brown the meat, stirring occasionally. Season with low sodium salt and pepper.
Add the chopped tomato, tomato sauce, and Italian seasoning and stir to combine. Simmer on low heat, stirring occasionally.
Add the sauce to the noodles and ENJOY.

69. Perfect Turkey Stir-Fry

Ingredients:
2 tbsp. of coconut oil
2 cloves of garlic (thinly sliced)
1 inch ginger (finely grated)
2-3 green (spring) onions (sliced into long slivers)
1 carrot (coarsely grated)
1 green pepper (sliced into thin, long pieces)
1 turkey breast (cut into bite-sized pieces)
1/4 cup water
2 tbsp. homemade veggie broth
A few drops of toasted sesame oil

Instructions:
Put a pot with a bit of low sodium salt to boil and make sure your rice noodles are handy. Later, when the water has boiled, pop the noodles in and give it a stir.
Heat 2 tbsp. coconut oil in a wok or large pan.
Add the sliced garlic and grated ginger to the wok and stir-fry for 30 seconds.
Add the green onion and stir-fry 1 more minute.
Add the carrot and stir-fry about a minute. You want it just barely cooked, not limp and soggy. Remove the vegetable mixture to a bowl and set aside.
Add another 2/3 tbsp. of coconut oil to the wok.
When the oil is very hot, add the green pepper and stir-fry for 1 minute.
Heat a ½ tbsp. of coconut oil, then add the pieces of turkey breast and stir-fry. I found that the turkey got some color from the previous ingredients that were in the wok. If this doesn't happen, add a tiny amount of soy sauce.
Stir-fry until just done and no more. To check, I like to cut open the biggest piece to make sure it isn't pink in the middle.
Add the sesame oil.

70. Creamy Curry Stir Fry

Ingredients:
2 cooked chicken breasts (small) or 3-4 thighs/legs
3 carrots, chopped
3 sticks celery, chopped
1-2 heads broccoli, chopped
1/2 medium onion, chopped
2 cloves garlic 1/2c coconut milk
1/2c almond or coconut milk
2 tbsp turmeric
2 tbsp curry powder
2 tbsp coconut oil

Instructions:
Put coconut oil in pan and add chopped onion. Cook until onion softens up, add garlic and cook for an additional few minutes.
Next up, add in the carrots, celery, and broccoli. Cook until they have softened a bit (but are not fully cooked).
Shred the cooked chicken up into small pieces for the stir fry and add the coconut milk, other milk, and curry spices.
Stir everything thoroughly, simmer for 5-10 minutes or until everything is cooked to your liking, and serve hot.
Add cauliflower rice (grated cauliflower boiled for 3 minutes)

71. Chicken Coconut Divine

Ingredients:
1 tbsp olive oil
1/2 tsp roasted cumin
1-1/2 tsp garam masala
2 tsp curry powder
1/2 onion, minced
5 cloves garlic, minced
1 large tomato, chopped
2 tbsp fresh cilantro, chopped
1/2 cup light coconut milk
3/4 cup water
6 skinless chicken thighs
Low sodium salt to taste

Instructions:
Add oil to a large pan, on medium heat. When oil is hot add onion and garlic and sauté.
Add cumin, masala and curry powder and mix well.
Place chicken in the pan and season with low sodium salt. Mix together with all spices and brown on both side for a few minutes.
Add tomatoes, cilantro, water, coconut milk and adjust low sodium salt to taste. Mix all ingredients and cover pan, simmer on low until chicken is cooked through, about 20 minutes.
Option ...Serve with Cauliflower rice

72. Coconut Turkey Salad

Ingredients:
6 (about 12 oz) turkey breasts
6 tbsp shredded coconut
Pinch low sodium salt
olive oil spray
6 cups mixed baby greens
3/4 cup shredded carrots
1 large tomato, sliced
1 small cucumber, sliced
2 beaten egg whites organic
For the Vinaigrette:
1 tbsp oil
Stevia to taste
1 tbsp white vinegar
2 tsp mustard powder
Instructions:
Whisk all vinaigrette ingredients; set aside.
Preheat oven to 375°.
Combine coconut flakes and low sodium salt in a bowl. Put egg whites or egg beaters in another bowl.
Lightly season chicken with low sodium salt. Dip the chicken in the egg, then in the coconut flake mixture. Place chicken on a cookie sheet lined with parchment for easy cleanup. Lightly spray with olive oil spray and bake for 30 minutes turning halfway, or until chicken is cooked through.
Place 2 cups baby greens on each plate. Divide carrots, cucumber, tomato evenly between each plate. When chicken is ready slice on the diagonal and place on top of greens. Heat dressing and divide equally between each salad; a little over 1 tbsp each.

73. Jolly Jamaican Chicken

Ingredients:
6 bone-in chicken legs with thighs attached, skin removed (6 thighs, 6 drumsticks)
1 lime or 1/4 cup lime juice
1 large tomato, chopped
4 medium scallions, chopped
1 large onion, chopped
2 garlic cloves, chopped
1/2 - 1 hot chilli, chopped
4 sprigs fresh thyme or 2 tsp dried thyme
2 tbsp low sodium soy sauce (for gluten free use GF Tamari)
1 tsp coconut oil 1 medium carrot, chopped finely
2 tsp almond flour
1 1/2 cups unsweetened light coconut milk
1/4 tsp low sodium salt

Instructions:
Squeeze lime over chicken and rub well. Drain off excess lime juice.

Using gloves combine tomato, scallion, onion, garlic, chilli pepper, thyme and soy sauce in a large bowl and add to the chicken. Cover and marinate at least one hour.

Heat oil in a large saucepan. Shake off the seasonings as you remove each piece of chicken from the marinade, reserving the marinade for later.

Lightly brown the chicken on medium-high heat. When browned on all sides, pour the marinade over the chicken and add the carrots. Stir and cook over medium heat for 10 minutes.

Mix flour and coconut milk and add to stew, stirring constantly. Reduce heat to low and cook an additional 20 minutes or until tender, add low sodium salt to taste.

74. Thai Baked Fish with Squash Noodles

Ingredients:
1 medium spaghetti squash
Extra virgin olive oil, for drizzling
low sodium salt and pepper
1 tbsp coconut oil
1/2 large onion, finely chopped
1 head broccoli, de-stemmed and cut into florets
2 heads baby bok choy, sliced into 1-inch strips
4 scallions, sliced
1/4 tsp red pepper flakes
1/3 cup cashews, toasted and chopped

For the Sauce:
1 tsp lime juice
1/2-inch piece fresh ginger, peeled and minced
1 clove garlic, minced
1/2 tsp red wine vinegar
3 tbsp almond butter
3 tbsp coconut milk

For the Fish:
2 whole fish fillets…use cod or any good quality white fish

Instructions:
Preheat the oven to 400 degrees F. Place squash in the microwave for 3-4 minutes to soften. Using a sharp knife, cut the squash in half lengthwise. Scoop out the seeds and discard. Place the halves, with the cut side up, on a rimmed baking sheet. Drizzle with olive oil and sprinkle with low sodium salt and pepper. Roast in the oven for 45-50 minutes, until you can poke the squash easily with a fork. Let cool until you can handle it safely. Then scrape the insides with a fork to shred the squash into strands.

While the squash cooks, make the sauce. Combine the lime juice, ginger, garlic, and red wine vinegar in a blender or food processor until smooth. Add the almond butter and coconut milk and blend until completely combined. Adjust the levels of almond butter and coconut milk to reach desired level of creaminess.

Melt the coconut oil in a large pan over medium heat. Add the onion and cook for 5-6 minutes until translucent. Add the broccoli and sauté for 8-10 minutes, until just tender. Then stir in the bok choy and cook for 3-4 minutes until wilted. Lastly add the cooked spaghetti squash into the pan and stir to combine.

To assemble, top the spaghetti squash mixture with the scallions and cilantro. Sprinkle with roasted cashews and drizzle with Thai sauce.

Place the whole fish under the grill at 200 degrees for 25 minutes topped with a tablespoon of olive oil, fresh pressed garlic (one clove) and cayenne pepper to taste.

Finnish off the fish with a squirt of lemon juice to taste.

75. Divine Prawn Mexicana

Ingredients:
1 tbsp extra virgin olive oil
1 tsp chili powder
1 tsp low sodium salt
1 lb. medium shrimp, peeled and deveined
1 avocado, pitted and diced
Shredded lettuce, for serving
Fresh cilantro, for serving
1 lime, cut into wedges
For the tortillas:
6 egg whites
1/4 cup coconut flour
1/4 cup almond milk
1/2 tsp low sodium salt
1/2 tsp cumin
1/4 tsp chili powder
Instructions:
Combine all of the tortilla ingredients together in a small bowl and mix well. Allow the batter to sit for approximately 10 minutes to allow the flour to soak up some of the moisture, and then stir again. The consistency should be similar to crepe batter.
While the batter is resting, heat a skillet to medium-high. Mix together the olive oil, chili powder, and low sodium salt and toss with the shrimp to coat. Cook in the skillet for 1-2 minutes per side, until translucent. Set aside.
Coat the pan with coconut oil spray. Pour about 1/4 cup of batter onto the skillet, turning the pan with your wrist to help it spread out in a thin, even layer. Cook for 1-2 minutes, loosening the sides with a spatula. When the bottom has firmed up, carefully flip over and cook for another 2-3 minutes until lightly browned, then set aside on a plate. Repeat with remaining batter.
Top each tortilla with cooked shrimp, shredded lettuce, avocado, and cilantro. Serve with a lime wedge.

76. Shrimp Cakes Delux

Ingredients:
2 cups of small prawns
2 eggs
fresh chives
1/2 tsp spicy chili powder
1/2 tsp ground coriander
1/2 tsp garlic powder
shredded coconut
1/2 tbsp coconut flour

Instructions:
In a saute pan over medium heat, warm the olive oil.
Add the garlic, red pepper flakes and paprika and saute for 1 minute until fragrant.
Increase the heat to high, add the shrimp, lime juice and sherry, stir well, and saute until the shrimp.
Season with low sodium salt and black pepper.

77. Shrimp Spinach Spectacular

Ingredients:
2 tablespoons olive oil
½ yellow onion – diced
1 cup green beans
2 cloves garlic minced
½ teaspoon chili powder
½ lime – juiced
1 pound raw wild shrimp – thawed, cleaned, and tails removed
1 – 6 oz. bag of baby spinach
low sodium salt and pepper to taste

Instructions:
Chop the shrimp,
Next, mix in the spices, chives, 1 egg and the coconut flour.
Set up 2 bowls, 1 with shredded coconut and the other with the 2nd egg, whisked.
Form cakes of the shrimp mix - cover them with the whisked egg and then with shredded coconut.
Cook them in coconut oil on both sides until brown.
Serve with vegetables of your choice, or fried cauliflower rice.

78. Turkey Eastern Surprise

Ingredients:
For the salad:
2 cups grilled turkey, chopped
6 baby bok choy, grilled & chopped
2 green onions, chopped
1/4 cup cilantro, chopped
1 Tbl sesame seeds
For the dressing:
1 Tbl fresh ginger, chopped
2 Tbl coconut cream
1 Tbl fish sauce
1 Tbl sesame oil
2 Tbl fresh lime juice
1 tsp stevia powder or to taste

Instructions:
Combine all of the salad ingredients until well mixed.
Add all of the ingredients for the dressing into a blender or food processor, and blend until mostly smooth – there may be some small chunks of ginger left, that's ok.
Pour the dressing over the salad and toss lightly until coated.
Garnish with more sesame seeds if desired.
 If possible let it sit for an hour in the fridge before serving so the flavors can really meld together.

79. Spaghetti Squash Hash Browns

Ingredients
1 cup spagetti squash threads from a roasted spaghetti squash
1 Tbs. butter, ghee, lard (real lard), or coconut oil
Sea salt, to taste
Instructions
Place the spaghetti squash threads in a clean kitchen towel and wring out as much water as possible over the sink. The squash will shrink in volume by about half.
Heat the oil/fat over medium-high heat in a sturdy skillet. Add the drained squash and compress with a spatula into an even layer over the bottom of the pan. Sprinkle the top with sea salt. Cook until golden brown, then flip. Sauté on the other side until crispy. Sprinkle with more salt and serve.

80. Super Tempting Tofu

INGREDIENTS
¼ cup hoisin sauce
1 tablespoon rice wine vinegar
2 teaspoon coconut aminos
1½ teaspoon hot chili paste
1½ teaspoon toasted sesame oil
12 ounces firm or extra firm pressed tofu, cubed
1 tablespoon extra virgin olive oil
2 tablespoons chopped cilantro
sesame seeds for sprinkling

INSTRUCTIONS
Combine hoisin sauce, rice wine vinegar, coconut aminos, hot chili paste and sesame oil in a small bowl. Mix until well combined and set aside.
Heat olive oil in a large skillet over medium high heat. Add half of the tofu and saute for 2 to 3 minutes, or until tofu starts to brown. Transfer browned tofu to a plate lined with paper towel to drain. Repeat with remaining tofu.
Add tofu back to skillet along with the hoisin mixture, tossing to coat tofu evenly.
Saute another 2 to 3 minutes, making sure tofu is evenly coated and sauce is throughly heated.
Remove from heat and serve over farro, rice, veggies, noodles, whatever you choose.
Sprinkle on sesame seeds and cilantro.
Serve and enjoy!

81. Crispy Baked Chicken Fingers

Ingredients
2 large skinless, boneless chicken breasts
1 cup almond meal/flour
¼ cup tapioca flour/starch
½ cup unsweetened shredded coconut
1 tsp garlic powder
1 tsp ground mustard powder
½ tsp smoked paprika
½ tsp sea salt
½ tsp ground black pepper
¼ tsp cayenne pepper
2 whole eggs, whisked
2-3 tbsp olive oil, for drizzling
Paleo Honey Mustard, for dipping

Instructions
Preheat oven to 400F. Line a baking sheet with parchment paper.
In a small bowl, whisk the eggs. Set aside.
Make your breading in a separate, larger bowl. To do this, whisk together the almond flour, tapioca flour/starch, unsweetened shredded coconut, garlic powder, ground mustard powder, smoked paprika, sea salt, ground black pepper and cayenne pepper.
Cut each of your chicken breasts into about 6 lengthwise strips, for a total of 12 strips. Place them all into your egg bowl.
One at a time, remove a chicken strip from the egg bowl and dip it in the "breading" mixture. Make sure to thoroughly coat all sides of the strip. Lay it on the parchment-lined baking sheet.
Once you've breaded all the strips, drizzle a little olive oil over the tops of each one – not too much, but not too little either!
Bake for a total of 17-20 minutes, depending on the size of your chicken fingers. Flip after 12-15 minutes of cooking time. (If the chicken fingers aren't looking golden or crispy enough at 20 minutes, turn up the heat to 425 and let them cook an additional 3 minutes.)
When the fingers are done, remove them from the oven and let them cool for a few minutes before serving with a side of Paleo Honey Mustard.
Store extra chicken fingers in an airtight container in the refrigerator for up to 3 days, or freeze for longer storage.

82. Balsamic Glaze Chicken Wings

Ingredients
1 cup water;
½ cup balsamic vinegar;
¼ cup coconut aminos (a Paleo-friendly replacement for soy sauce; you can get them online or at most health-food stores);
¼ cup honey;
1 tsp. Sriracha sauce; (optional or to taste)

Preparation

Mix up the marinade by combining the honey, if using, coconut aminos, lime juice, garlic powder, curry powder, ginger powder, and Chinese 5 spice powder in a bowl. Season to taste with salt and pepper.

Add the chicken to the marinade and marinate for a minimum of 4 hours and up to overnight in the refrigerator.

Preheat your oven to 400 F.

Line a baking sheet with parchment paper and place the chicken wings on top.

Bake on the middle rack of your oven for 40 minutes.

While the wings are cooking, combine the glaze ingredients in a skillet and let simmer for 10 to 15 minutes, or until the glaze is sticky. If you're using sriracha sauce, stir it in at the last minute.

Turn your oven to broil and broil for approximately 5 minutes or until crispy.

Remove the chicken wings from the oven and transfer to a large bowl.

Add the glaze with the chicken wings, toss to coat, and serve.

19. Orange and Miso Glazed Salmon

2 skinless salmon fillets (weighing approximately 150 grams each)

the glaze

1 tablespoon white miso

juice of one orange (approximately 1/2 cup)

2 teaspoons honey

Heat a medium sized frypan over medium heat.

Add the glaze ingredients to the frypan and stir to combine.

Bring the glaze to a gentle boil. Add the salmon fillets. Reduce the heat to a simmer. Cook for 5 minutes, turn and cook for a further 5 minutes. You may want to increase the heat slightly to get a nice caramelisation on the salmon.

Serve with salad or vegetables of your choice.

Enjoy.

83. Zucchini Fritters

Ingredients
2 Zucchini (grated)
1 tsp Sea salt
2 tbsp Coconut flour
4 Scallions (sliced)
1 Egg
1 tsp Cayenne pepper
1 tsp Black pepper
2 tbsp Coconut oil

Instructions
In a medium-sized mixing bowl, stir together the shredded zucchini and sea salt. Set aside for 10 minutes.
After 10 minutes, squeeze the water out of the zucchini and transfer to a clean bowl.
Stir in the coconut flour, egg, scallions, cayenne, and pepper.
Add the coconut oil to a medium skillet over medium-high heat.
Once the coconut oil has melted, form six fritters and place them in the skillet. Brown on each side then set aside on a paper-towel lined plate.
Serve immediately. Garnish with additional scallions.

84. Sundried Tomato Roulade

Ingredients
4 Turkey cutlets
6-7 Sundried tomatoes
3 tbsp Fresh basil leaves (about 20 leaves)
2 tbsp Pine nuts
1/2 tsp Sea salt
3-4 tbsp olive oil
Sea salt and black pepper (to taste)
Coconut oil

Instructions
Preheat the oven to 350 degrees F.

Place a skillet over medium-high heat. Add the pine nuts to toast. Toast in the dry pan for 3 to 4 minutes shaking occasionally so they don't stick. Do not leave unattended, they can burn quickly.

Using a food processor or blender, blend together the sun-dried tomatoes, basil, toasted pine nuts, and salt until well combined. Drizzle the olive in while processing.

Lay each cutlet out on your work surface. Season with salt. Then spread the sun-dried tomato mixture on the surface of each cutlet

Start at one end and tightly roll the cutlet and secure with a toothpick.

Add the coconut oil to an oven-proof medium skillet over medium-high heat.

Add each roulade to the hot skillet, browning on each side. Use soft-tipped tongs to turn so you don't damage the meat.

Place in the preheated oven for another 10 minutes, or until each is cooked through.

Use a sharp knife to cut into roulade discs. Season to taste.

Enjoy!

85. Beefy Shanky Broth

INGREDIENTS:

2 lbs/1 kilo beef shanks (I choose bones about 2"- 2-1/2" diameter). The meat is completely optional, but I find it a nice benefit. If you prefer to cook bones only, use 2 lbs of bones.
1-2 liters cold, filtered water
4 Tbsp Apple Cider Vinegar
2 Bay Leaves
2 Tbsp Sea Salt, divided (or 3 Tbsp Magic Mushroom Powder)
2 Tbsp Tamari, Fish sauce, coconut aminos OR Worcestershire sauce (always opt for gluten free)
1 tsp Garlic, granulated
1 tsp dried Oregano
2 tsp dried Parsley
1 tsp dried Thyme
1 cup Onions (white or yellow), sliced
1 cup Carrot, sliced in rounds
1/2 cup Celery, sliced
1 Tbsp butter, ghee or coconut oil (for the seering pan)
Optional: 1/2 cup sliced mushrooms (button or shitake)

INSTRUCTIONS:

Heat butter, ghee or coconut oil in a large frying pan or griddle over med-high heat. Add the beef shanks to the pre-heated pan, along with 1 Tbsp sea salt and the dried spices (garlic, oregano, parsley and thyme) and cook for 4-5 minutes per side or until a nice brown crust starts to form on the meat. Turn the meat and cook the other side for an additional 3-4 minutes.

86. Coconut Crusted Baked Cauliflower Bites

Ingredients
1/2 cup all-purpose flour
1/2 teaspoon salt
1/2 teaspoon garlic powder
1/2 teaspoon onion powder
1 egg
1/2 cup Silk coconut milk
1/2 cup Panko breadcrumbs
1/2 cup sweetened coconut flakes
1 head cauliflower (roughly 2 pounds), cut into small florets
Marinara Sauce
1 tablespoon olive oil
1/2 cup chopped onion
1 clove garlic, minced
1 can (14 ounces) diced tomatoes with juices
1 teaspoon sugar
1 teaspoon dried basil
1 teaspoon dried oregano
1 teaspoon dried parsley
1/4 teaspoon salt
Instructions

Preheat oven to 450F. Line the bottom of a roasting pan or cookie sheet with foil. Place a roasting or cooling rack on top. Lightly spray the rack with cooking spray.
In a shallow plate or bowl, whisk together the flour, salt, garlic powder, and onion powder. In a second plate or bowl, whisk together the egg and coconut milk. In a third plate or bowl, mix together the breadcrumbs and coconut flakes.
Dip one cauliflower floret into the flour mixture then the coconut milk mixture then the breadcrumb mixture. Place on the rack. Repeat until all of the cauliflower is gone.
Bake 15-20 minutes or until golden brown. Serve with marinara dipping sauce (recipe below)
Marinara Dipping Sauce
In a large saucepan, heat the olive oil until hot. Add the onion and cook until soft, about 5 minutes. Add the garlic and cook 30 seconds. Add the tomatoes with juices, sugar, basil, oregano, parsley, and salt. Bring to a boil. Once boiling, cover and simmer for 15 minutes. Add the sauce to a blender and blend until smooth. Serve with cauliflower bites.

87. Crockpot Maple and Balsamic Glazed pork Loin

Ingredients:
1-2 lb pork tenderloin
2 tsp ground sage
1/2 tsp salt
1/4 tsp pepper
1 garlic clove, minced
1/4 – 1/2 cup of water (use 1/4 if you have a 1lb tenderloin, 1/2 if it is 2 lbs)
For the glaze:
3 tbsp maple syrup
1/4 cup balsamic vinegar
1 tbsp cornstarch
2 tbsp coconut aminos (or low-sodium soy sauce)
Directions:
Combine sage, salt, pepper and garlic in a small bowl. Prepare loin by trimming any fat and patting dry with paper towels. Rub the sage mixture over all sides of the pork. Place in crock pot with 1/4-1/2 cup water. Cook on low for 6-8 hours.
About 1 hour before roast is done, whisk together ingredients for glaze in small sauce pan. Heat and stir until mixture thickens. Brush the pork with the glaze 2 or 3 times during the last hour of cooking. Serve with remaining glaze on the side.
6-10 servings. 21 Day Fix: measure out with your red container and count as one red serving.

88. Cauliflower Buffalo Bites

Ingredients
1 large head cauliflower, cut into bite-size florets
Olive oil to drizzle
2 teaspoons garlic powder
¼ teaspoon salt
⅛ teaspoon pepper
1 tablespoon melted butter (Use coconut oil for vegan option)
½ to *3/4 cup Frank's Buffalo Wing Style hot sauce or other hot wing sauce of choice
Other: 1 gallon or larger size plastic bag
*I probably use about ⅔ cup of hot sauce and they have just enough heat.

Instructions
Preheat oven to 450F degrees.
Place cauliflower florets into plastic bag. Drizzle olive oil over florets to barely coat.
Add garlic powder, salt and pepper. Close bag and toss ingredients around so all florets are coated.
Place on ungreased cookie sheet or baking pan and bake on middle rack for 15 minutes, turning florets once during baking. Check them at the 10 minute mark for desired tenderness. You don't want them to be soggy!
Remove florets from oven. Melt butter in medium glass bowl. Add hot sauce to butter. Toss cauliflower and stir to cover all florets with hot sauce. Start with about half the sauce and add more to your taste.
Return to oven and cook for additional 5 minutes.
Serve with any dip you like, ranch dressing or Blue Cheese dip.

89. Spicy Steak

Ingredients:
For Steak
2 pounds skirt steak
1/3 cup soy sauce
1/4 cup chili sesame oil
1 tablespoon mirin
3 tablespoons rice vinegar
1 lime, juiced
3 tablespoons of minced ginger
1 tablespoon of minced garlic
1 tablespoon siracha
1 tablespoon of toasted sesame seeds for garnish
1 tablespoon coconut oil
 For Slaw
1 head of purple cabbage, shredded
1 red pepper, diced
1 yellow pepper, diced
1 cucumber diced
2 tablespoons soy sauce
1 lime, juiced
2 tablespoon rice wine vinegar
1 tablespoon apple cider vinegar
2 tablespoons minced ginger
1 teaspoon peanut butter
2 teaspoons brown sugar
2 tablespoons sesame oil
3 tablespoons toasted sesame seeds

Directions:

For marinade, combine soy sauce, chili sesame oil, mirin, rice vinegar, lime juice, ginger, garlic, brown sugar, and siracha in a non reactive casserole dish and whisk together. Add steak and allow to marinate for 20 to 30 minutes while you prepare slaw. For slaw, mix shredded cabbage, red peppers, yellow peppers, and cucumber in a bowl. In a separate bowl, whisk together soy sauce, lime juice, rice wine vinegar, apple cider vinegar, ginger, peanut butter, brown sugar, sesame oil and sesame seeds. Pour dressing over vegetables and mix well. Allow slaw to cool in fridge while you prepare steak. Heat large skillet over medium high heat. Add 1 tablespoon of coconut oil. Remove skirt steak from marinade and cook for 5-6 minutes on each side for medium. Allow steak to rest for 5 minutes before slicing and serving.

90. Dark Chocolate

Ingredients
1/2 cup coconut oil (105 grams)*
1 cup unprocessed cocoa powder or cacao powder (118 grams)
4 tablespoons honey or more for taste
1 teaspoon pure vanilla extract**
pinch of sea salt

Instructions

Begin by melting the coconut oil in a small pot over the stove top on a low heat.

Once melted remove the oil from the heat and add the cocoa powder, honey, vanilla, sea salt and any additional flavors you want to add.

Whisk everything completely until there are no remaining lumps of cocoa powder and the honey has dissolved into the chocolate mixture.

Pour the chocolate into silicone molds or a lined baking pan and transfer to the freezer for at least 30 minutes or in the fridge for at least an hour. Once they've hardened pop them out of the molds and enjoy.

91. Totally Tahini Cups

INGREDIENTS:
1/3 cup (80 g) tahini
1/3 cup (79 ml) melted coconut oil
INSTRUCTIONS:
Combine the ingredients by hand or in a food processor until smooth. It will be a bit watery but the coconut oil will harden up in the fridge. Pour half of the mixture into the bottom of 6 cupcake liners and put in fridge for 20 minutes, or until solid. Set aside the other half of the tahini mixture.

92. Pumpkin crepes

ingredients
Apple Butter:
apples - 5 lb, peeled and sliced
cinnamon - to taste
Crepes:
egg yolk - 1
egg whites - 4
pure pumpkin puree - 1/3 cup
canned full-fat coconut milk - 1/3 cup
coconut flour - 3-4 tablespoons
arrowroot starch - 1/4 cup
pure vanilla extract - 1 teaspoon
ground allspice - 1/4 teaspoon
pure maple syrup - 3 tablespoons
instructions
Preheat oven to 425 degrees Fahrenheit.
Combine the apples and cinnamon to taste on 2 9 inch by 13 inch baking dishes.
Roast for 1-2 hours, stirring every 15 minutes, or until the apples have lost quite a bit of moisture.
Puree until smooth, adding water if necessary.
Preheat a nonstick skillet to 350 degrees Fahrenheit. Whisk together all crepe ingredients in a large bowl until smooth.
Lightly grease the skillet with coconut oil and add 4-5 tablespoons of batter, spreading it around with the back of a spoon.
Cook until the batter looks dry. Flip and cook until golden. Repeat with remaining batter.
Serve crepes with apple butter.

93. Lemon Cookies

Ingredients:
2 cups blanched almond flour
1/4 cup coconut flour
1/2 cup granulated sugar
1 teaspoon baking powder
1/8 teaspoon salt
1/2 cup unsalted butter, melted and cooled slightly
1 large egg, room temperature
1 tablespoon lemon zest (from 1 lemon)
1 teaspoon lemon extract
1/3 cup lemon curd*
powdered sugar, optional

Directions:
In a medium mixing bowl, stir together the almond flour, coconut flour, sugar, baking powder and salt. Set aside.
In another medium mixing bowl, stir together the melted butter, egg, lemon zest, and lemon extract.
Add the dry mixture to the wet and stir just until combined. The dough will feel quite wet. Let it sit for 10 minutes to allow the coconut flour to absorb the liquid while the oven preheats.
Preheat the oven to 350 degrees F and line a cookie sheet with a piece of parchment paper.
Roll the dough into 1" balls and place 2" apart on the prepared cookie sheet. The dough will feel quite greasy.
Bake the cookies for 6 minutes and remove from the oven.
Using the rounded part of a 1/2 teaspoon measuring spoon, make an indentation about 3/4 of the way down into each cookie.
Fill each indentation with 1/2 teaspoon of lemon curd. Be sure not to overfill them.

Return the pan to the oven and bake for another 5-7 minutes or until the cookies feel like they have a firm outer layer. The cookies shouldn't brown around the edges - just on the bottom.
Let the cookies, which will be very soft at this point, cool for 5 minutes on the baking sheet and then remove to a wire rack to cool completely. The parchment paper may be a little greasy, but the cookies will not be.
10. Refrigerate in an airtight container for up to 4 days. Dust with powdered sugar before serving, if desired.

Notes:
I've never seen lemon curd containing gluten but if you eat gluten-free, please check the ingredients label on your jar to ensure that your lemon curd doesn't have gluten.

94. Banana Shake

Ingredients
1 frozen banana, sliced
1/2 cup ice cubes
1/2 cup strong coffee**
2 tablespoons cocoa powder

1 tablespoon coconut butter (optional)
small splash of vanilla extract (optional)
Instructions:
Place all ingredients in a blender and process until smooth.
Makes approximately 1 serving

95. Spectacular Spinach Omelet

Ingredients:
2 eggs
1.5 cups raw spinach
coconut oil, about 1 tbsp
1/3 c tomatoes and onion salsa (lightly fried in pan)
1 tbsp fresh cilantro

Instructions:
Melt coconut oil on medium in frying pan. Add spinach, cook until mostly wilted. Beat eggs and add to pan.
Flip once the egg sets around the edge. When it's almost done add the salsa on top just to warm it. Move to plate and add cilantro. Serves one.

96. Blushing Blueberry Omelet

Ingredients:
2 eggs
1 tsp. vanilla extract
coconut oil
1/2 c. blueberries
Stevia to taste

Instructions:
Lightly beat two eggs and vanilla extract in a bowl. Heat 6" non-stick pan over medium heat.
While pan is heating, heat half the blueberries in a saucepan until juices flow.
Add coconut oil to non-stick pan and coat evenly.
When thoroughly heated, add egg mixture. Swish once and let sit.
When eggs are about 70% settled, swish again. There should be a nice crispy layer around the side of the pan.
When it starts to separate from the side, add fresh and cooked blueberries to omelet, reserving a few for garnish.
Crispy layer should really be pulling away from pan now.
 Use a fork to help fold the omelet over. Slide on to plate, top with reserved blueberry filling, and enjoy

97. Roasted and Filled Tasty Bell Peppers

Ingredients:
5 large bell peppers
1 tbsp coconut oil
1/2 large onion, diced
1 tsp dried oregano
1/2 tsp low sodium salt
1 lb. ground turkey
1 large zucchini, halved and diced
3 tbsp tomato paste
Freshly ground black pepper, to taste
Fresh parsley, for serving

Instructions:
Preheat the oven to 350 degrees F. Coat a small baking dish with coconut oil spray. Bring a large pot of water to a boil. Cut the stems and very top of the peppers off, removing the seeds. Place in boiling water for 4-5 minutes. Remove from the water and drain face-down on a paper towel.

Heat the coconut oil in a large nonstick pan over medium heat. Add in the onion. Sauté for 3-4 minutes until the onion begins to soften. Stir in the ground turkey, oregano, low sodium salt, and pepper and cook until turkey is browned.

Add the zucchini to the skillet as the turkey finishes cooking. Cook everything together until the zucchini is soft, and then drain any juices from the pan.

Remove the pan from heat and stir in the tomato paste. Bake for 15 minutes.

98. Creamy Chicken Casserole

Ingredients:
2 cups cubed cooked chicken
1 1/2 cups cooked butternut squash
1/2 cup coconut cream,
1/4 cup coconut oil, melted
1 heaping cup green peas, fresh or frozen
1 tbsp apple cider vinegar
1/2 tsp low sodium salt
1/2 tsp oregano
1/2 tsp thyme
1 tbsp fresh parsley
Instructions:
In a large bowl, mash the butternut squash. Stir in the coconut cream, oil, vinegar, low sodium salt, oregano, and thyme.
Once everything is combined, add in chicken and peas.
Place the mixture into a large saucepan and cook over medium heat for 5-8 minutes.
Top with fresh parsley and serve warm.

99. Ostrich Steak or Venison with Divine Mustard Sauce and Roasted Tomatoes

Ingredients:
For the tomatoes:
2 pints cherry tomatoes, halved
2 tbsp extra virgin olive oil
Stevia to taste
low sodium salt and freshly ground pepper
For the cauliflower rice:
1/2 head of cauliflower, chopped coarsely
1/2 small onion, finely diced
1 tbsp coconut oil
1 tbsp fresh parsley, chopped
low sodium salt and freshly ground pepper, to taste
For the meat:
4 Ostrich or venison steaks
Extra virgin olive oil
low sodium salt and freshly ground pepper
Coconut oil, for the pan
For the sauce:
1/4 cup red onion, finely diced
1/4 cup apple cider vinegar
1 cup low sodium chicken stock
1 tbsp whole grain mustard
low sodium salt and freshly ground pepper, to taste

Instructions:

Preheat the oven to 400 degrees F. Place the tomatoes on a baking sheet and drizzle with olive oil and honey. Sprinkle with low sodium salt and pepper and toss to coat evenly. Bake for 15-20 minutes until soft.

While the tomatoes are roasting, prepare the cauliflower rice. Place the cauliflower into a food processor and pulse until reduced to the size of rice grains.

Melt the coconut oil in a nonstick skillet over medium heat. Add the onion and cook for 5-6 minutes until translucent. Stir in the cauliflower, season with low sodium salt and pepper, and cover. Cook for 7-10 minutes until the cauliflower has softened, and then toss with parsley.

To make the lamb, preheat the oven to 325 degrees F. Pat the ostrich or venison dry and rub with olive oil. Generously season both sides with low sodium salt and pepper.

Heat one tablespoon of coconut oil in a cast iron skillet. When the pan is hot, add to the pan and sear for 2-3 minutes on all sides until golden brown.

Place the skillet in the oven and bake for 5-8 minutes until the ostrich or venison reaches desired doneness. Let rest for 10 minutes before serving.

While the meat is resting, add the red onion to the skillet with the pan drippings from the lamb. Sauté for 3-4 minutes, then add the white wine vinegar.

Turn the heat to high and cook until the vinegar has mostly evaporated. Add the stock and bring to a boil, cooking until the sauce reduces by half.

Stir in the mustard, and season to taste with low sodium salt and pepper. Pour over ostrich or venison to serve.

100. Tantalizing Turkey Pepper Stir-fry

Ingredients:
2 bell peppers, sliced
1 cup broccoli florets
2 cooked and shredded turkey breasts
1/4 teaspoon chili powder
low sodium salt and pepper to taste
1 tablespoon coconut oil for frying

Instructions:
Add 1 tablespoon coconut oil into a frying pan on a medium heat.
Place the sliced bell peppers into the frying pan.
After the bell peppers soften, add in the cooked turkey meat.
Add in the chili powder, low sodium salt and pepper.
Mix well and stir-fry for a few more minutes.

101. Cheeky Chicken Stir Fry

Ingredients:
1 pound boneless, skinless chicken breast
2 tablespoons coconut oil
1 medium onion, finely chopped (about 1 cup)
2 heads broccoli, sliced into 3-inch spears (about 4 cups)
2 medium carrots, sliced (about 1 cup)
2 heads baby bok choy, sliced crosswise into 1-inch strips (about 1½ cups)
4 ounces shiitake mushrooms, stemmed and thinly sliced (about 1 cup)
1 small zucchini, sliced (about 1 cup)
½ teaspoon low sodium salt
Garlic powder to taste
1½ cups water

Instructions:
Rinse the chicken and pat dry. Cut into 1-inch cubes and transfer to a plate.
Heat the coconut oil in a large skillet over medium heat
Saute the onion for 8 to 10 minutes, until soft and translucent
Add the broccoli, carrots, and chicken and saute for 10 minutes until almost tender
Add the bok choy, mushrooms, zucchini, and low sodium salt and saute for 5 minutes
Add 1 cup of the water, cover the skillet, and cook for about 10 minutes, until the vegetables are wilted
In a small bowl, dissolve the arrowroot powder in the remaining ½ cup of water, stirring until thoroughly combined
Season at the end with garlic powder, salt and if you like some chilli powder

102. Turkey Thai Basil

Ingredients:
2 lbs. leftover cooked turkey, cubed or shredded (chicken or shrimp would work too)
3 Tbsp fish sauce
3 Tbsp coconut aminos (or wheat free tamari)
1 Tbsp water
Stevia to taste
1 tsp low sodium salt
1/2 tsp ground white pepper
2 Tbsp coconut oil
4 baby bok choy, leaves pulled apart, hearts halved
1 red bell pepper, sliced
1 yellow bell pepper, sliced
1 large onion, sliced
3 cloves garlic, minced
1 1/2 C lightly pack Thai basil leaves

Instructions:
In a medium bowl, combine turkey with fish sauce, water, low sodium salt and pepper; stir until turkey is thoroughly coated and set aside
Melt coconut oil in large wok or frying pan over medium-high heat
Add bok choy, peppers, onion and garlic and saute until softened, about 8 minutes, stirring frequently
Add contents of set-aside bowl (with the meat) to pan and stir for about 3 minutes until turkey is fully incorporated and heated through
Remove from heat and add Thai basil, stirring until basil wilts

103. Chicken Fennel Stir-Fry

Ingredients:
3 chicken breasts or the meat from 1 whole roasted chicken
2 tablespoons coconut oil
1 onion
1 bulb of fennel
1 teaspoon each of low sodium salt, pepper, garlic powder and basil

Instructions:

Stovetop:

Cut the chicken into bite sized pieces. If chicken is raw, heat butter/coconut oil in large skillet or wok until melted.

Add chicken and cook on medium/high heat until chicken is cooked through. (If chicken is pre-cooked, cook the vegetables first then add chicken)

While cooking, cut the onion into bite sized pieces (1/2 inch) and thinly slice the fennel bulb into thin slivers.

Add all to skillet or wok, add spices and continue sautéing until all are cooked through and fragrant.

This will take approximately 10-12 minutes.

104. Prawn garlic Fried "Rice"

Ingredients:
1 tbsp coconut oil
1 cup white onion, finely chopped
2 cloves garlic, minced
8 oz. prawns peeled and deveined
1 medium carrot, chopped
1/2 cup peas
2 cups cooked cauliflower rice
2 eggs, beaten
Low sodium salt and pepper, to taste

Instructions:
Heat a wok or large pan over medium-high heat. Melt the coconut oil and add the onion and garlic to the pan.
Cook for 3-4 minutes until the onion starts to soften. Add the shrimp and cook for 1 minute.
Add the carrot, peas, and bell pepper to the pan. Cook for 3-4 minutes, and then stir in the cauliflower rice.
Clear a circle in the center of the pan and pour in the beaten eggs. Stir to scramble the eggs and then combine with the other ingredients.
Season with low sodium salt and pepper to taste.

105. Lemon and Thyme Super Salmon

Ingredients:
32 oz piece of salmon
1 lemon, sliced thin
2 tspns lemon juice
Low sodium salt and freshly ground pepper
1 tbsp fresh thyme
Olive oil, for drizzling

Instructions:
Heat a wok or large pan over medium-high heat. Melt the coconut oil and add the onion and garlic to the pan.
Cook for 3-4 minutes until the onion starts to soften. Add the shrimp and cook for 1 minute.
Add the carrot, peas, and bell pepper to the pan. Cook for 3-4 minutes, and then stir in the cauliflower rice.
Clear a circle in the center of the pan and pour in the beaten eggs. Stir to scramble the eggs and then combine with the other ingredients.
Season with low sodium salt and pepper to taste.

106. Spectacular Spaghetti and Delish Turkey Balls

Ingredients:
1 spaghetti squash
Extra virgin olive oil,
low sodium salt and pepper
1 tsp dried or fresh oregano
For the sauce:
1 lb ground turkey
1 small onion, chopped
4 cloves garlic, minced
1 tbsp coconut oil
1 tomato, chopped
1/2 jar of tomato sauce
1 tbsp Italian seasoning
low sodium salt and pepper to taste
Fresh basil

Instructions:
Preheat oven to 400 degrees F. Using a sharp knife, cut the squash in half lengthwise. Scoop out the seeds and discard. Place the halves with the cut side up on a rimmed baking sheet. Drizzle with olive oil and season with low sodium salt, pepper, and oregano. Roast the squash in the oven for 40-45 minutes, until you can poke the squash easily with a fork.
Let it cool until you can handle it safely. Then scrape the insides with a fork to shred the squash into strands.
While the spaghetti squash is roasting, melt coconut oil in a large skillet over medium heat.
Add chopped onion and garlic and cook for 4-5 minutes. Add ground turkey and brown the meat, stirring occasionally. Season with low sodium salt and pepper.
Add the chopped tomato, tomato sauce, and Italian seasoning and stir to combine. Simmer on low heat, stirring occasionally, while the spaghetti squash finishes roasting. Serve over spaghetti squash with basil for garnish.

107. Prawn Salad Boats

Ingredients:
1 lb shrimp, cooked
1 medium tomato, diced
1 cucumber, peeled and diced
3 tablespoons olive oil
One tablespoon coconut cream
Juice of one lemon
1/2 tsp dried dill
1/2 tsp celery seed
1/4 tsp low sodium salt
1/4 tsp pepper
Endive or big lettuce leaf, for serving

Instructions:

In a large sauté pan, heat olive oil over medium heat. Add onion, beans, and sauté until tender –approximately 10 minutes.

Add garlic, lime juice, and chili powder and continue to cook for an additional 5 minutes.

Add spinach and shrimp. Continue to cook for approximately 7-10 more minutes until spinach has wilted and shrimp is done.

108. Sexy Shrimp with Delish Veggie Stir Fry

Ingredients:
1 1/2 pounds of shrimp
1 tsp. of coconut oil
1/2 cup of thinly sliced onion
1/2 red bell pepper. thinly sliced
1 cup of full fat coconut milk
2 tbsp. fish sauce
1 tbsp curry powder
2 tbsp. of chopped cilantro

Instructions:
In a large bowl mix fish sauce, garlic and ginger.

Heat the olive oil in a wok (or a large nonstick skillet) over medium-high heat.

Once it starts to shimmer add onion and chiles. Stir-fry the onions until they start to brown around the edges, about 2 minutes.

Stir in the bok choy stems and stir-fry for 1 minute.

Add the beaten eggs and cook until it's nearly cooked through about 2 minutes, stirring often.

Stir in bok choy greens, basil and lime juice. And stir-fry for 30 seconds or so, until the greens are wilted. Serve immediately.

109. Peachy Prawn Coconut

Ingredients:
1 1/4 lbs jumbo prawns, peeled and deveined (weight after peeled)
1 tsp extra virgin olive oil
1 red bell pepper, sliced thin
4 scallions, thinly sliced, white and green parts separated
1/2 cup cilantro
4 cloves garlic, minced
Low sodium salt (to taste)
1/2 tsp crushed red pepper flakes (to taste)
14.5 oz can diced tomatoes
14 oz can light coconut milk (50% less fat)*
1/2 lime, squeezed

Instructions:
In a medium pot, heat oil on low. Add red peppers and sauté until soft (about 4 minutes).
Add scallion whites, 1/4 cup cilantro, red pepper flakes and garlic. Cook 1 minute.
Add tomatoes, coconut milk and low sodium salt to taste, cover and simmer on low about 10 minutes to let the flavors blend together and to thicken the sauce.
Add prawns and cook 5 minutes. Add lime juice.
To serve, divide equally among 4 bowls and top with scallions and cilantro.
Serve with cauliflower rice

110. Rosy Chicken Supreme Salad

Ingredients:
For the chicken:
450g chicken mince, free range of course
1 long red chili, finely chopped with the seeds
2 garlic cloves, finely chopped
Little nob of fresh ginger, peeled and finely chopped
1 stem lemon grass, pale section only, finely chopped
1/2 bunch of coriander stems washed and finely chopped (I don't waste anything, save the leaves for the salad)
2 1/2 tbsp fish sauce
1/2 lime rind grated
1/2 lime, juiced
A pinch of low sodium salt
Coconut oil for frying (about 3 tablespoons)
For the salad:
1/4 red cabbage, thinly sliced
1 large carrot, peeled and grated
1/2 Spanish onion, thinly sliced
2 tbsp green spring onion, chopped
1/2 bunch of fresh coriander leaves (saved from the stems used in the chicken)
A handful of fresh mint or Thai basil if available
1/2 cup crashed roasted cashews or some sesame seeds
For the dressing:
2 tbsp olive oil
3 tbsp lime juice
1 tbsp fish sauce
1 small red chili, finely chopped
Instructions:
Once you've prepared all your ingredients for the chicken, heat 1 tbsp of coconut oil in a large frying pan or a wok to high.
Throw in lemongrass, chili, garlic, coriander stems and ginger and stir fry for about a minute until fragrant.
Add chicken mince and lime zest. Stir and break apart the mince with a wooden mixing spoon until separated into small chunks (this might take a while as chicken mince is quite sticky).
The meat will now be changing to white colour.
Add fish sauce and lime juice. Stir through and cook for a further few minutes. Total cooking time for the chicken should be about 10 minutes.
Prepare the salad base by mixing together sliced red cabbage, onion grated carrot, and fresh herbs.
Mix all dressing ingredients and toss through the salad.
Serve cooked chicken mince on top of the dressed salad and topped with roasted cashews, dried shallots, coconut flakes and extra fresh herbs.

111. Creamy Carrot Salad

Ingredients:
1 pound carrots - shredded
20 ounces crushed pineapple -- drained
8 ounces Coconut milk
3/4 cup flaked coconut
Stevia to taste
Shredded turkey one breast
Instructions:
Combine all ingredients, tossing well. Cover and chill.

112. Quick And Easy Broth

INGREDIENTS
Bones from 1 or 2 chickens (feet if possible), or 2-3 lbs of beef bones
1-2 onions
4-5 garlic cloves
rosemary or thyme (optional)
2 tablespoons coconut vinegar (or apple cider vinegar)
Salt to taste
Just enough water to cover all ingredients

INSTRUCTIONS
Place all ingredients in a large stockpot and bring to a boil.
Reduce to simmer and cook on low for 8 hours minimum, but as long as possible. I like to start it in the morning and let it cook all day.
Once done cooking, remove the bones and let cool to use again. Once cool, place in a gallon zip bag and freeze.
Place a fine mesh strainer over a large bowl and carefully pour the broth through the strainer. Discard all the solid bits.
Cover and refrigerate overnight.
Once fully cooled, a layer of fat will be on the top. I always remove it and throw it away, but that is optional.
Divide into mason jars and store in the fridge.
This can also be frozen. I like freezing it in a mini muffin tin, then once frozen, putting them in a quart size bag. This makes adding them to dishes very easy.

113. Turkey Stockbroth

Ingredients
2 tablespoons coconut oil
1 medium onion, diced
2 cloves garlic, minced
1 pound turkey BONES
1 tablespoon coconut amino
10 cups chicken broth
1/4 teaspoon salt
1/4 teaspoon pepper
4 cups fresh spinach leaves, coarsely chopped
Fresh rosemary, optional
Directions
Heat the coconut oil in a large stockpot over high heat. Add the onion and garlic and sauté for 2 minutes. Add the ground turkey and sauté for an additional 7 minutes.
Add the coconut amines. Stir frequently for 2 minutes.
Add the chicken broth, salt, and pepper. Simmer for about 20 minutes.
Add the spinach and rosemary (if desired) and sauté for 2 minutes.

114. Simple Beef and Broccoli Stir Fry

Ingredients
1.5 lbs. sirloin, thinly sliced
4 tbsp coconut aminos, divided
4 tbsp red wine vinegar, divided
3 tbsp chicken broth
4 cloves garlic, minced
1 tsp arrowroot flour
1 tsp honey
1 tbsp ginger, minced
1/2 tsp sesame oil
1 head broccoli, cut into florets
4 carrots, diagonally sliced
3 tbsp coconut oil, divided

Instructions

Place the sirloin in a small bowl with one tablespoon each of red wine vinegar and coconut aminos and toss to coat. Let marinate for 15 minutes at room temperature.

Meanwhile, whisk together 3 tablespoons each red wine vinegar, coconut aminos, and chicken broth. Stir in the garlic, ginger, arrowroot, honey, and sesame oil. Prepare a separate small bowl with 1 tablespoon of water and set it next to the stove along with the garlic sauce.

Melt 2 tablespoons of coconut oil in a large skillet over medium heat. Place the steak in the skillet in a single layer. The meat should sizzle; otherwise the pan is not hot enough. Cook for 1-2 minutes per side to brown, and then transfer to a bowl.

Add the remaining tablespoon of coconut oil to the skillet. Stir in the broccoli and carrots, cooking for 2 minutes. Add the water to the skillet and cover with a lid. Let cook for 2-3 minutes, then remove the lid and cook until all of the water has evaporated.

Add the garlic mixture to the vegetables and stir to coat. Add the beef back into the pan and toss until the sauce thickens and everything is well coated. Serve immediately.

Notes
Servings: 4-6
Difficulty: Medium

115. Homemade Sweet and Salty Paleo Granola

Ingredients
1 cup cashews
3/4 cup almonds
1/4 cup pumpkin seeds, shelled
1/4 cup sunflower seeds, shelled
1/2 cup unsweetened coconut flakes
1/4 cup coconut oil
1/4 cup honey
1 tsp vanilla
1 cup dried cranberries
1 tsp salt
Instructions
Preheat oven to 300 degrees F. Line a baking sheet with parchment paper. Place the cashews, almonds, coconut flakes and pumpkin seeds into a blender and pulse to break the mixture into smaller pieces.

In a large microwave-safe bowl, melt the coconut oil, vanilla, and honey together for 40-50 seconds. Add in the mixture from the blender and the sunflower seeds, and stir to coat.

Spread the mixture out onto the baking sheet and cook for 20-25 minutes, stirring once, until the mixture is lightly browned. Remove from heat. Stir in the dried cranberries and salt.

Press the granola mixture together to form a flat, even surface. Cool for about 15 minutes, and then break into chunks. Store in an airtight container or resealable bag.

Notes
Servings: 6
Difficulty: Easy

116. Curry Coconut Salad

Ingredients:
6 large ripe tomatoes, peeled, seeded and chopped
1 small white onion, grated
1/4 tsp. coarsely ground pepper
1/2 cup coconut cream
2 Tbsp minced fresh parsley
1 tsp. curry powder

Instructions:
Combine tomatoes, onion and pepper; cover and chill for 3 hours.
Combine coconut cream, parsley and curry; cover and chill for 3 hours.
To serve, spoon tomato mixture into small bowls and top each with a spoonful of coconut cream mixture.

117. Prawn garlic Fried "Rice"

Ingredients:
1 tbsp coconut oil
1 cup white onion, finely chopped
2 cloves garlic, minced
8 oz. prawns peeled and deveined
1 medium carrot, chopped
1/2 cup peas
2 cups cooked cauliflower rice
2 eggs, beaten
Low sodium salt and pepper, to taste

Instructions:
Heat a wok or large pan over medium-high heat. Melt the coconut oil and add the onion and garlic to the pan.
Cook for 3-4 minutes until the onion starts to soften. Add the shrimp and cook for 1 minute.
Add the carrot, peas, and bell pepper to the pan. Cook for 3-4 minutes, and then stir in the cauliflower rice.
Clear a circle in the center of the pan and pour in the beaten eggs. Stir to scramble the eggs and then combine with the other ingredients.
Season with low sodium salt and pepper to taste

118. Creamy Carrot Salad

Ingredients:
1 pound carrots - shredded
20 ounces crushed pineapple -- drained
8 ounces Coconut milk
3/4 cup flaked coconut
Stevia to taste
Shredded turkey one breast
Instructions:
Combine all ingredients, tossing well. Cover and chill.

119. Skinny Chicken salad

Ingredients:
Salad:
1 small head (or 4 cups) savoy cabbage, finely shredded –
1 cup carrot, julienned
1/4 cup scallions, trimmed and julienned
1/4 cup radishes, julienned
1/4 cup fresh cilantro, chopped
1/4 cup fresh mint, chopped
2 cups cooked organic chicken
Vinaigrette:
2 tablespoons coconut or rice vinegar
2 tablespoons sesame oil (use unrefined, expeller or cold-pressed)
juice of 1/2 a lime
1 chipotle pepper (or sub
1 clove garlic, crushed
1 teaspoon fresh ginger, grated

Instructions:
Salad – Combine cabbage, carrots, scallions and radishes. Top with chicken, cilantro and mint and set aside.
Vinaigrette –Combine the vinaigrette ingredients. Taste to see if it needs any adjustments. If it is too spicy, you can add more lime juice to counteract it.
Drizzle salad with vinaigrette & enjoy.

120. Spectacular Spinach Omelet

Ingredients:
2 eggs
1.5 cups raw spinach
coconut oil, about 1 tbsp
1/3 c tomatoes and onion salsa (lightly fried in pan)
1 tbsp fresh cilantro

Instructions:
Melt coconut oil on medium in frying pan. Add spinach, cook until mostly wilted. Beat eggs and add to pan.
Flip once the egg sets around the edge. When it's almost done add the salsa on top just to warm it. Move to plate and add cilantro. Serves one.

121. Blushing Blueberry Omelet

Ingredients:
2 eggs
1 tsp. vanilla extract
coconut oil
1/2 c. blueberries
Stevia to taste

Instructions:
Lightly beat two eggs and vanilla extract in a bowl. Heat 6" non-stick pan over medium heat.
While pan is heating, heat half the blueberries in a saucepan until juices flow.
Add coconut oil to non-stick pan and coat evenly.
When thoroughly heated, add egg mixture. Swish once and let sit.
When eggs are about 70% settled, swish again. There should be a nice crispy layer around the side of the pan.
When it starts to separate from the side, add fresh and cooked blueberries to omelet, reserving a few for garnish.
Crispy layer should really be pulling away from pan now.
 Use a fork to help fold the omelet over. Slide on to plate, top with reserved blueberry filling, and enjoy

Paleo Diet Recipes 365 Days of Paleo and Coconut Recipes by Mercedes Del Rey

122. Paleo Shrimp Fried "Rice"

Ingredients
1 tbsp coconut oil
1 cup white onion, finely chopped
2 cloves garlic, minced
8 oz. shrimp, peeled and deveined
1 medium carrot, chopped
1/2 cup peas
1/4 cup red bell pepper, finely chopped
2 cups cooked cauliflower rice
2 eggs, beaten
Salt and pepper, to taste

Instructions
Heat a wok or large pan over medium-high heat. Melt the coconut oil and add the onion and garlic to the pan. Cook for 3-4 minutes until the onion starts to soften. Add the shrimp and cook for 1 minute.

Add the carrot, peas, and bell pepper to the pan. Cook for 3-4 minutes, and then stir in the cauliflower rice. Clear a circle in the center of the pan and pour in the beaten eggs. Stir to scramble the eggs and then combine with the other ingredients. Season with salt and pepper to taste.

Notes
Servings: 2
Difficulty: Easy

123. Asparagus Quiche with Spaghetti Squash Crust

Ingredients
1 medium spaghetti squash (use about 2 1/2 – 3 cups of the meat for this recipe)
2 tablespoons butter
1 large leek, thinly sliced
3 tablespoons butter
5 large eggs, beaten
1 cup coconut milk/almond milk/dairy milk (I used almond milk, as that's all that we had left)
a bunch of thin asparagus (about 2 cups), cut in halves or large pieces
1 medium tomato, cut in thin slices and then halve the slices
sea salt and freshly ground pepper, to taste
1/2 – 1 teaspoon ground nutmeg

Instructions
Preheat the oven to 375F (190C).
Carefully split the spaghetti squash in half. (It can also be baked whole, but it will take longer.)
Remove the seeds and sprouts, if any, with hands.
Place cut-side down on a baking pan.
Bake for 40 minutes, or until tender.
In the meantime, poach the asparagus in some water, until just tender. Remove from water and set aside.
Allow the spaghetti squash to cool a bit before removing the meat with a fork.
Mix about 2 1/2 to 3 cups of the meat with 2 tablespoons of butter and mix well.
Add sea salt and pepper, to taste. (Remember that the egg mixture will also contain seasoning, so don't go overboard.)
Pat the squash into a quiche form, covering the sides and bottom.
Bake at 400F (200C) for about 5-8 minutes, until golden and slightly crispy. Remove from oven and set aside.
In a saucepan, over medium heat, cook the leek slices with the 3 tablespoons butter, until tender.
Allow to slightly cool before pouring into the beaten eggs.
Add the milk, nutmeg, sea salt and pepper to taste.
Place the poached asparagus pieces on top of the spaghetti squash crust.
Pour the beaten eggs and leeks over top, covering the asparagus evenly.
Place the tomato pieces on top.
Bake for 35-40 minutes.

124. Garden Pea, Feta & Mint Tart

Garden Pea, Feta & Mint Tart (serves 6-8)
Crust:
1/2 cup butter, melted
2 large eggs
3/4 cup coconut flour
1/2 tsp sea salt

Instruction
Whisk together the eggs and butter.
Sieve the coconut flour into a large mixing bowl. Add the salt.
Gradually add the wet ingredients to the dry and mix until it forms a soft batter.
Press this into a greased 9in pie dish. It won't cooperate like regular dough, that's ok. Just press it in with your hands until the dish is covered. Prick the base.
Bake at 375 for 5 minutes. Remove and let cool while you sort out the filling.
Filling:
4oz feta cheese, crumbled
1 1/2 cups peas (I used frozen and defrosted beforehand)
2 spring/green onions, finely chopped
2 tbsps fresh mint leaves, chopped
3 large eggs
1/2 cup plain yoghurt
salt and pepper
Instructions
Whisk the eggs, yoghurt and seasoning together. Stir in the peas, feta and onions.
Fold in the mint and pour the whole mixture into your pie crust.
Bake at 375 for 25-30 mins till firm. Let cool for a few minutes before slicing up.

Paleo Diet Recipes 365 Days of Paleo and Coconut Recipes by Mercedes Del Rey

125. Garlicky Collard Pie

Ingredients
2 tablespoons ghee, butter or lard
1 small yellow onion, diced
4 cloves garlic, minced
4 cups collards or other hearty greens, rinsed and chopped
1 1/2 teaspoons kosher or sea salt
3/4 teaspoon freshly-ground black pepper
2 ounces pecorino romano or other hard Italian cheese, shredded
10 large eggs
3/4 cup coconut milk plus 1/2 cup water or 1 1/4 cups half and half
2 teaspoons garlic powder
1 teaspoon dried thyme
1 teaspoon dried oregano

Instructions
Preheat the oven to 375 F. Generously grease a 10" deep-dish pie plate with butter or non-hydrogenated palm oil shortening.
Melt the ghee in a large, heavy skillet over medium heat. Cook the onion until soft and almost translucent, about 5 minutes; add the garlic and cook for another minute more. Add the collard greens and cook, stirring frequently, until they are wilted. Season with the salt and pepper and remove from the heat.
In a large bowl, whisk together the eggs with the water, coconut milk, garlic powder, thyme and oregano until well blended. Spread the collard/onion mixture over the bottom of the greased pie plate; sprinkle the cheese evenly over the greens. Carefully pour the egg mixture over the cheese and greens.
Bake the pie for 25 to 35 minutes, or until the top is golden brown and a knife inserted in the center comes out clean.
Cool for 30 minutes before cutting into wedges. Serve with a chunky salsa or warm marinara sauce.
Nutrition (per serving): 203 calories, 15.5g total fat, 247.5mg cholesterol, 534.7mg sodium, 210.4mg potassium, 5.2g carbohydrates, 1.1g fiber, <1g sugar, 11.3g protein.

126. Crustless Broccoli and Sausage Quiche

1. 1 medium onion, chopped
2. 1 pound of bulk sausage (just remove casings if you can't find it in bulk)
3. 2 cloves of garlic, grated
4. coconut oil
5. 12 oz. of broccoli
6. 10 eggs
7. sea salt/pepper/TJ's 21 seasoning salute

Instructions:

Preheat your oven to 350 degrees. saute the onion in coconut oil over medium-highish heat.

season with salt, pepper and 21 salute. once the onions are cooked halfway (translucent and soft) add the sausage meat. crumble the sausage as it cooks.

As the sausage is cooking, liberally grease a 9 x 13 pan in coconut oil. i suggest a small sandwich bag over your hand so you don't miss any spots or corners. next, in a large bowl, whisk the eggs vigorously. season with salt and pepper.

The broccoli i used was frozen in one of the steam-ready bags you throw into the microwave. instead of cooking it for 5 minutes in the microwave, i cooked it for only 2 so it was defrosted but not cooked all the way through. if you are using fresh broccoli, i would suggest blanching it for a minute or 2, any longer than that and it might get mushy. add the broccoli to the sausage mixture and cook for a minute or two.

Finally, add the garlic to the sausage mixture, cook for one additional minute and then remove from the heat. place the broccoli-sausage mixture into the greased baking dish. pour the eggs over the top of the meat and vegetables and bake uncovered for 25-30 minutes.

127. Bacon and Tomato Quiche

Ingredients
Zucchini Hash Crust:
2 small to medium size organic zucchini, grated
1 egg, beaten
1 1/2 Tbsp coconut flour
1 tsp flax meal *optional
1 tbsp butter or coconut oil melted
1/8 tsp sea salt

Quiche:
5 eggs, beaten
1/2 cup organic egg whites, (I used the ones in a carton, but make sure egg white is the only ingredient) or you could separate 3 eggs
3 Tbsp milk of choice: organic heavy cream, or unsweetened plain almond milk
5 slices nitrate free bacon, cooked and chopped (make sure bacon has no sugar in the ingredients)
2/3 cup cauliflower, ground into rice (you won't taste it, and it adds nutrients and fiber)
1/2 cup fresh spinach, chopped * optional
1/4 tsp ground mustard
1/4 tsp sea salt (I use Real Salt or Himalayan sea salt)
1/4 tsp black pepper
Topping:
2 small to medium sized tomatoes, sliced (I used 6 slices).
1/2 cup grated cheese of choice * optional
Instructions
Preheat oven to 400 F, and grease or oil pie dish.
Grate or use processor on zucchini.
Wrap grated zucchini in layered paper towels or cheese cloth. Squeeze and drain liquid from zucchini over sink. Place drained zucchini in large bowl.
Add all the remaining crust ingredients to the zucchini and mix together.
Place zucchini mixture into pie dish. Use the back of a spoon to spread mixture around pie dish, until dish is covered in zucchini crust mixture.
Bake zucchini crust in oven for 9 minutes.
Remove crust from oven (leave oven on). Set aside.
In large mixing bowl combine: eggs, egg whites, milk of choice, ground mustard, sea salt, and black pepper.
Grate or use processor on the cauliflower until rice texture forms.
Add cauliflower rice, chopped spinach, and chopped bacon to the egg mixture and combine.
Pour egg mixture into zucchini crust.
Place tomato slices on top of quiche.
Bake for 28 minutes, but check at 20 minutes to see if crust edges are browning too much.
Loosely cover the top of pie dish with a parchment paper sheet. Place back in oven for remaining 8 minutes, or until top is browned and center is firm and set.
Add optional cheese and put back in oven for 2 minutes.
Remove and let cool.
Slice and serve.
Notes

Net Carb Count*: 8.15 g net carbs (per 1 slice - makes 8 slices)
Total Carb Count: 11.79 g total carbs (per 1 slice - makes 8 slices)

128. Paleo Turkey Pesto Meatballs

Ingredients
2 lbs. ground turkey
1/2 cup almond flour
1/2 cup pesto
2 egg whites
1/2 tsp salt
1/4 tsp freshly ground pepper
Instructions
Preheat the oven to 375 degrees F. Line a baking sheet with aluminum foil and then place a wire cooling rack on top of the baking sheet. Coat the wire rack well with coconut oil spray.
In a large bowl, mix together all of the ingredients. Roll the mixture into small balls using your hands and place on the wire rack. Bake for 20-25 minutes until cooked through.
Notes
Servings: 24 meatballs
Difficulty: Easy

129. Broccoli Egg Bake (So Wholesome & Healthy)

Ingredients
8 eggs
1/2 large onion, diced
2 medium zucchini, diced
1 medium head of broccoli, chopped
1 tsp salt
1/2 tsp freshly ground black pepper
1 tbsp fresh parsley, chopped
Instructions
Preheat the oven to 350 degrees F. In a small bowl, whisk the eggs, salt and pepper. Stir in the chopped vegetables. Grease a ramekin with coconut oil spray. Pour egg mixture into the dish and bake for 25-30 minutes or until the eggs are set. Remove from heat and let sit for 5 minutes before serving. Top with chopped parsley to serve.
Notes
Servings: 6
Difficulty: Easy

130. Meatball Sandwich with Zucchini "Bread" & Coconut Curry Sauce

Meatballs
½ onion
½ tomato
4 cloves of garlic
1 egg
2 tbsp coconut milk
2 tsp sea salt
½ tsp black pepper
½ tsp paprika
1 lb. of grass-fed ground beef.
Zucchini "bread" and coconut sauce
1 onion
1 tomato
3 cloves of garlic
250g can coconut milk
4 very large zucchinis or 8 small ones (one per sandwich)
1 tsp sea salt
1 tsp curry powder
1 lemon
Parsley
Instructions
Preheat your over to 350 degrees. Line two roasting trays with aluminum foil.
Dice your tomato, onion and garlic. Set aside.
For the meatballs, crack open your egg and mix in tomato, onion, garlic, salt, black pepper and coconut milk.
It's time to get intimate with your creation. Put your beef into a mixing bowl and using your hands knead in the egg mixture. Shape into lovely little meatballs and place on roasting tray and put tray into heated oven for 20 minutes.
While your meatballs form into edible creations take your washed zucchini and slice them in half. Then dig out about 1/3 of the zucchini meat on one half and ½ from the top half.
Dice up the zucchini meat and add onion, tomato, garlic, salt, curry powder and add the coconut cream only (the water on the bottom is not needed so use it tomorrow for a tasty addition to a Crockpot chicken soup).
Mix everything and pour into your waiting zucchini tunnels. Remove your meatballs from the oven and place your zucchini into the oven at the same temperature.
Cook your guys for 20 minutes uncovered and then cover them with a sheet of foil for another 10 minutes.
Chop up your parsley and lemon wedges for plating.
Remove zucchini from oven and sprinkle some lemon juice on top. Nestle the meatballs into the deeper zucchini half place your second zucchini half on top, slice in half and serve with some parsley and lemon on the side for a mini salad garnish.
Notes
You can use a knife and fork but for sandwich-style eating wrap the bottom halves of your sandwiches in wax paper (the red and white checkered kind if you can get it) so you can hold on to your grub and have a delightful conversation at the same time.

131. Spicy Steak

Ingredients:
For Steak
2 pounds skirt steak
1/3 cup soy sauce
1/4 cup chili sesame oil
1 tablespoon mirin
3 tablespoons rice vinegar
1 lime, juiced
3 tablespoons of minced ginger
1 tablespoon of minced garlic

1 tablespoon siracha
1 tablespoon of toasted sesame seeds for garnish
1 tablespoon coconut oil

For Slaw
1 head of purple cabbage, shredded
1 red pepper, diced
1 yellow pepper, diced
1 cucumber diced
2 tablespoons soy sauce
1 lime, juiced
2 tablespoon rice wine vinegar
1 tablespoon apple cider vinegar
2 tablespoons minced ginger
1 teaspoon peanut butter
2 teaspoons brown sugar
2 tablespoons sesame oil
3 tablespoons toasted sesame seeds

Directions:
For marinade, combine soy sauce, chili sesame oil, mirin, rice vinegar, lime juice, ginger, garlic, brown sugar, and siracha in a non reactive casserole dish and whisk together. Add steak and allow to marinate for 20 to 30 minutes while you prepare slaw. For slaw, mix shredded cabbage, red peppers, yellow peppers, and cucumber in a bowl. In a separate bowl, whisk together soy sauce, lime juice, rice wine vinegar, apple cider vinegar, ginger, peanut butter, brown sugar, sesame oil and sesame seeds. Pour dressing over vegetables and mix well. Allow slaw to cool in fridge while you prepare steak. Heat large skillet over medium high heat. Add 1 tablespoon of coconut oil. Remove skirt steak from marinade and cook for 5-6 minutes on each side for medium. Allow steak to rest for 5 minutes before slicing and serving.

132. Easy Homemade Gluten-Free Energy Bars

Ingredients
1 cup almonds
1 cup dried cranberries
1 cup pitted dates
1 tbsp unsweetened coconut flakes
1/4 cup mini dark chocolate chips
Instructions
Combine all of the ingredients in a blender or food processor. Pulse a few times to break everything up. Then blend continuously until the ingredients have broken down and start to clump together into a ball.
Using a spatula to scrape down the sides, turn out the mixture onto a piece of wax paper or plastic wrap. Press into an even square and chill, wrapped, for at least an hour. Cut into desired size of bars, wrapping each bar in plastic wrap to store in the fridge.
Notes
Servings: 8 bars
Difficulty: Easy

133. Gummi Orange Slices

Ingredients:
1 T. vanilla extract
½ t. natural orange flavour
Pinch real salt
1 ½ t. liquid stevia (every brand varies in sweetness, so add this 'to taste')
8 T. grass-fed gelatin
1 can coconut milk
1 ½ C. water
Natural orange food colouring to desired colour
orange ice cube tray molds

INSTRUCTIONS:
Heat water and coconut milk over low heat until simmering.
Continue on low heat, slowly adding in each tablespoon of gelatin, whisking the entire time.
Add remaining ingredients and whisk until any clumps of gelatin are gone.
Pour into molds, and pour remaining liquid into 8X8 glass pan.
Put in fridge until solid. Gummis should pop out easily once hardened.

134. Spicy Steak

Ingredients:
For Steak
2 pounds skirt steak
1/3 cup soy sauce
1/4 cup chili sesame oil
1 tablespoon mirin
3 tablespoons rice vinegar
1 lime, juiced
3 tablespoons of minced ginger
1 tablespoon of minced garlic

1 tablespoon siracha
1 tablespoon of toasted sesame seeds for garnish
1 tablespoon coconut oil

For Slaw
1 head of purple cabbage, shredded
1 red pepper, diced
1 yellow pepper, diced
1 cucumber diced
2 tablespoons soy sauce
1 lime, juiced
2 tablespoon rice wine vinegar
1 tablespoon apple cider vinegar
2 tablespoons minced ginger
1 teaspoon peanut butter
2 teaspoons brown sugar
2 tablespoons sesame oil
3 tablespoons toasted sesame seeds

Directions:
For marinade, combine soy sauce, chili sesame oil, mirin, rice vinegar, lime juice, ginger, garlic, brown sugar, and siracha in a non reactive casserole dish and whisk together. Add steak and allow to marinate for 20 to 30 minutes while you prepare slaw. For slaw, mix shredded cabbage, red peppers, yellow peppers, and cucumber in a bowl. In a separate bowl, whisk together soy sauce, lime juice, rice wine vinegar, apple cider vinegar, ginger, peanut butter, brown sugar, sesame oil and sesame seeds. Pour dressing over vegetables and mix well. Allow slaw to cool in fridge while you prepare steak. Heat large skillet over medium high heat. Add 1 tablespoon of coconut oil. Remove skirt steak from marinade and cook for 5-6 minutes on each side for medium. Allow steak to rest for 5 minutes before slicing and serving.

135. Baked Sweet Potato Chips

Ingredients
2 large sweet potatoes
2 tbsp melted coconut oil
2 tsp dried rosemary
1 tsp sea salt
Instructions
Preheat oven to 375 degrees F. Peel sweet potatoes and slice thinly, using either a mandolin or sharp knife. In a large bowl, toss sweet potatoes with coconut oil, rosemary, and salt.

Place sweet potato chips in a single layer on a rimmed baking sheet covered with parchment paper. Bake in the oven for 10 minutes, then flip the chips over and bake for another 10 minutes. For the last ten minutes, watch the chips closely and pull off any chips that start to brown, until all of the chips are cooked.

136. Gummi Orange Slices

Ingredients:
1 T. vanilla extract
½ t. natural orange flavour
Pinch real salt
1 ½ t. liquid stevia (every brand varies in sweetness, so add this 'to taste')
8 T. grass-fed gelatin
1 can coconut milk
1 ½ C. water
Natural orange food colouring to desired colour
orange ice cube tray molds

INSTRUCTIONS:
Heat water and coconut milk over low heat until simmering.
Continue on low heat, slowly adding in each tablespoon of gelatin, whisking the entire time.
Add remaining ingredients and whisk until any clumps of gelatin are gone.
Pour into molds, and pour remaining liquid into 8X8 glass pan.
Put in fridge until solid. Gummis should pop out easily once hardened.

137. Prosciutto-Wrapped Berries

Yields: 12 total strawberries/baby bell peppers
6 strawberries
6 golden baby bell peppers
Honey Basil Ricotta (see below)
1 oz. thinly sliced grass-fed proscuitto, divided into 12 strips
1/4 c. micro greens (about half a small package)
Instructions
Using a sharp pairing knife, cut the tops off the strawberries, pulling the middle completely out and leaving a deep hole. Do the same for the peppers and use your finger to pull any seeds out of the insides.

To assemble: use a butter knife to stuff the berries/peppers with about 1 t. each of the Honey Basil Ricotta (the peppers will hold more ricotta than the berries). Then place a few sprigs of micro greens into the ricotta. Wrap a thin slice of proscuitto around each one and lay down length-wise to hold the proscuitto in place (you could also use toothpicks for this but that's a little too fussy for me).

138. Vanilla Pumpkin Seed Clusters

Ingredients:
115g (1/2 cup) pumpkin seeds
1 tsp vanilla extract
2 tsp honey
2 tsp coconut sugar
Water (boiled)

Instructions

Preheat oven to 150c.

In a medium bowl, combine the honey, coconut sugar and vanilla. Stir together to create a thick paste then add a small drop of boiled water to thin it out and create a runny syrup.

Pour in the pumpkin seeds and stir them around in the mixture to evenly coat them.

Dollop a generous tsp full of the pumpkin seeds onto a baking sheet, repeat until it's all used up and cook for 15-20 minutes until most of the seeds have browned (but don't let them burn!)

Take out of the oven and leave to cool for a few minutes. Once they've cooled a little (but are still warm) you can press the clusters together to make sure they don't fall apart. They will dry quickly.

Once they're cooled and dried, they're ready to eat! Enjoy on their own or served on top of your cereal.

139. Almond Joy Sunday

Ingredients:
1. 2 cans full fat coconut milk
2. ½ cup honey
3. 1 ½ tablespoons vanilla extract
4. 1 dark baking chocolate bar
5. ¼ cup sliced almonds
6. ½ cup unsweetened coconut flakes

Instructions

1. In a blender, mix together the coconut milk, honey, and vanilla extract. Line a plastic Tupperware with plastic wrap. Pour the mixture into it and freeze it overnight. The next day, take half of the frozen mixture and add it to a food processor. Mix it on high until it resembles frozen yogurt and put it back into a storage container. Repeat this process with the other half of the mixture. Return the blended ice cream to the freeze for 30 minutes before serving.

2. To assemble, melt the chocolate chips in a saucepan over low heat, to prevent burning the chocolate. Serve each Almond Joy Sunday with a scoop of the ice cream. Drizzle the melted chocolate on top, then sprinkle with coconut flakes and sliced almonds. Serve immediately.

140. Spiced Autumn Apples Baked in Brandy

Ingredients
2 apples of your choice (I used gala, but choose your favourite!)
1 cup brandy
1/4 cup walnuts
1/4 cup raisins
1/4 tablespoon nutmeg
1/4 tablespoon cinnamon
1/4 tablespoon ground cloves

Directions
Preheat oven to 350 degrees Fahrenheit.
Slice the very top and very bottom off of each apple. (The top allows for more room to stuff with goodies, the bottom allows the apples to soak up all the nice sauce).
Core both apples to the bottom, but not all the way through.
Mix brandy, spices, walnuts, and raisins in a small bowl.
Pour half of the brandy spice mixture into each apple.
Place on baking sheet and bake 20-25 minutes, or until apples are soft. I like to pour any remaining sauce mixture into the bottom of the pan so the apples can soak up the flavours.
Serve and enjoy! My roommate enjoyed his with a side of vanilla coconut milk ice cream.

Notes
Recipe makes 2 servings
Nutrition Facts Per Serving
Calories: 353
Total Fat: 10.0g
Saturated Fat: 0.6g
Carbs: 32.4g
Fiber: 4.0g
Protein: 4.6g

141. Chocolate Bavarian Cheesecake

Ingredients:
For the base:
15 Easy Chocolate Cookies
¼ cup coconut oil (melted)
OR
2 cups nuts
2. 1 cup dried dates (soaked in water)
For the middle:
2+1/2 cups raw cashews (soaked in water for 6 or more hours)
½ cup honey
¼ cup coconut oil
¼ cup cacao powder
½ cup coconut milk
½ cup orange juice
For the top:
1 can coconut cream (chilled in fridge overnight)
Cacao nibs to decorate

Instructions:
For the base:
Grind the chocolate cookies in a food processor until fine. Add the melted coconut oil and process until mixture sticks together. Add another tablespoon of coconut oil if you need to.
Press the crumbs into the base of a 21cm springform tin. If you don't have a springform tin, just line your tin with plastic wrap or baking paper so you can remove it easily.
OR
If you can't be bothered making the cookies (or didn't have any in the freezer like I did), just process 2 cups of nuts in a food processor until finely chopped. (Any combination of nuts works well. I've tried just macadamias and it is beautiful and also a combination of cashews, macadamias, hazelnuts, walnuts and brazil nuts)
When your nuts are finely chopped, drain the soaked dates, getting out as much water as you can. Then add them to the food processor and process until it makes a sticky dough.
Next, scoop the date & nut mixture into your pan. Put small plastic freezer bags onto your hands and use your fingers to spread the mixture evenly into the pan. (No sticky fingers!)
For the filling:
Drain the cashews well. Put all of the filling ingredients into a high speed blender or processor and process until smooth. I have a new Froothie blender that is amazing! I compared it to the Vita Mix and it's cheaper and more powerful. You know I love a bargain. Anyway, I'm really happy with it and it makes amazing cheesecake filling!
You will need to use the tamper if you have one and regularly scrape down the sides to make sure all the ingredients are blended together. Keep processing until it is super smooth. Lots of taste testing needed for this step!
Once the mixture is smooth, scrape it all into your pan, on top of the base mixture. Spread it out with a spatula.
Cover with plastic wrap, then put into the freezer for at least 6 hours to set.
When ready to serve, take it from the freezer and defrost for around 30 minutes to soften slightly before cutting. (15 mins for minis.)
While it's defrosting, beat the cream that rises to the top of the coconut cream after it's been refrigerated. Use electric beaters and add some honey to taste if you like.
Spread or pipe the cream over the top of your cheesecake and decorate with cacao nibs.

142. Maple Cinnamon Cheesecakes with Gingerbread Crust

Ingredients
For the crust:
1 heaping cup pecans
6 medjool dates
½ tsp ginger
½ tsp cinnamon
For the cheesecake:
2 cups raw cashews (soaked overnight)
½ cup maple syrup
½ tsp cinnamon
Juice of 1 lemon
⅓ cup coconut oil
½ tsp sea salt

Instructions

For the crust:
Combine all the ingredients in a food processor. You will see the mixture start to get to a crumbly like consistency. Be careful not to over process or you will end up with pecan butter. Once the mixture looks done, you can press a little into the bottom of each muffin cup. I used standard sized pans. Place them in the fridge while you make the cheesecake part.
For the cheesecake:
Make sure your cashews have been soaking overnight. Drain and rinse them. Place them in a food processor with all the other cheesecake ingredients. Mix until everything is smooth.
Spoon a little of the cheesecake mixture into each muffin cup.
Once that is done, place them in the fridge to firm up. It can take up to 12 hours for the cheesecakes to get fully firm.
Notes
Keep these stored in the fridge. You can probably freeze them as well. I have not tried that though.

143. Heavenly Raw Vegan White Chocolate and Raspberry Cheesecake

Ingredients
Base layer:
1 cup almonds
6 medjool dates, pitted
2 tbsp cocoa butter, liquified
¼ tsp raw ground vanilla beans (or ½ tsp pure vanilla extract)
Cheesecake layer:
1½ cups cashews, pre-soaked (at least a few hours, best overnight) and strained
¼ cup fresh squeezed lemon juice
6 tbsp liquid sweetener of your choice (I used maple syrup)
¼ cup coconut oil, liquified
⅓ cup cocoa butter, liquified
1 tsp pure vanilla extract (or ½ tsp more ground raw vanilla bean)
¼ tsp salt
Raspberry topping layer:
1½ – 2 cups fresh or frozen raspberries (I used frozen and slightly thawed out)
3 tbsp liquid sweetener or your choice (I used maple syrup)
⅓ cup cocoa butter, liquified
Optional:
Reserve a few raspberries for garnish
Instructions
Place all base ingredients into a food processor and process until a medium-fine crumbly mixture is formed. Transfer this mixture into the springform pan and press down well to create an even flat cake base. Place in the freezer while working on the next step (or for at least 10 minutes).

Place all cheesecake layer ingredients in your blender (a stronger blender like a Vitamix works best), and blend until mixture is completely smooth. Pour it over the crust into the springform pan. Lightly tap the pan down on the counter to eliminate any air bubbles. Smooth it out as well to create an even surface. Place in the freezer while working on the next step (best if in the freezer for at least 15 – 20 minutes). {Placing cake in the freezer for a bit helps keep the cake layers better separated}

Place all raspberry layer ingredients into your blender and blend until the mixture is smooth. Pour over the cheesecake layer into the springform pan and return back to the freezer for at least 3-4 hours. Cake can then be served out of the freezer as an icebox cake, or kept refrigerated for a softer and more mousse-like consistency. I kept mine frozen, but allowed it to thaw out for about an hour in the fridge before serving. Decorate with some fresh raspberries prior to serving and enjoy!

144. Samoa Donuts

Ingredients
For the Donuts
2½ cups blanched almond flour (such as Honeyville)
½ teaspoon baking soda
A scant less than ½ teaspoon salt
6 tablespoons honey
¼ cup coconut oil, softened or liquid
1 tablespoon vanilla
1 teaspoon Lemon juice
3 whole large room temp eggs
Coconut caramel topping
1 can full-fat coconut milk (about 1½ cups), I used guar gum-free Natural Value
½ cup mild flavored honey or maple syrup,
A pinch of sea salt
1 rounded tablespoon ghee or butter (can sub palm shortening or coconut oil)
2 teaspoons vanilla extract
¼ cup finely shredded coconut, plus 2 more tablespoons for garnishing
For the Dipping Chocolate
1 bag Enjoy Life Chocolate chips (melted in a double boiler)
Instructions
Preheat your mini donut making machine OR preheat the oven to 350 degrees if you are using a regular donut pan or making into muffins.
In a large bowl, mix together the almond flour, baking soda and salt.
In another bowl, combine the honey, oil, vanilla, lemon juice and eggs.
Add the oil/honey mixture to the dry ingredients. Mix till just combined.
Add about 2 tablespoons of batter to each mould in the donut machine or scoop the batter into a ziplock bag, twisting the other end to close it. Snip the end off of one of the corners with a scissors. Start with a small cut. You can always make it bigger if you need too. Squeeze batter into moulds.
Close the lid and allow to cook for about 2 minutes. Times will vary with each machine. Open the machine and flip over each donut using the forked 'skewer' that comes with most machines. Close the lid again cook for about one more minute. Remove donuts and let cool on a wire rack. Repeat with the rest of the batter.
If using a regular donut pan, fill each well-greased mould about ¾ full. Smooth the tops if needed and bake for 10-12 minutes. Let cool in the pan for 5 minutes, remove from the pan and cool completely on a wire rack.
Makes 12-15 mini donuts or 6 regular sized ones (depending on how much batter you eat during the prep time.)
For the Coconut Caramel
In a small-medium heavy bottomed sauce pan, bring the coconut milk, honey and salt to a boil over medium high heat, being sure that they are well combined. Reduce to a medium heat, and let the mixture boil down for about 35-40 minutes. Add the ghee and vanilla, stirring it in till well incorporated. Continue cooking for another 5-15 minutes or as long as needed until it is a deep caramel color. Don't rush the process. Depending on how hot your burner is this process could be faster or slower. Stir often toward the end to keep the bottom from burning too much. A little burning is fine as long as you are stirring it in to the mixture. It will give it a darker flavor.
Remove from heat, transfer to a bowl and let cool for 5 minutes then stir vigorously until it's creamy, shinny and smooth.
While the caramel is cooking, spread the coconut out on an ungreased cookie sheet and toast the coconut in a 325 degree oven. Stir often till golden, about 5-10 minutes. Remove from the oven and let cool.

Mix the toasted coconut into the caramel minus a tablespoon or so for garnishing later. Use coconut caramel while still warm for best spreading results. Caramel can be made ahead of time(w/o the shredded coconut) and reheated in a double boiler.

145. Hummingbird Bread

Ingredients
½ cup tapioca flour/powder
½ cup coconut flour
½ cup coconut sugar
½ teaspoon cinnamon
½ teaspoon baking soda
pinch of salt
2 bananas, mashed
½ cup pineapple, diced
½ cup coconut oil, melted
3 eggs, whisked
1 teaspoon vanilla extract
½ cup pecans, chopped
Instructions
Preheat oven to 350 degrees.
Add tapioca flour, coconut flour, coconut suguar, cinnamon, baking soda, and salt to a large bowl and mix. Then add the rest of the ingredients, folding in pecans at the end.
Pour mixture into a bread pan (I lined mine with parchment paper for easy removal) and smooth at the top
Bake for 40-45 minutes or until bread is completely cooked through (use the toothpick trick to check)
Let cool slightly before serving.

146. Earl Grey Lavender Ice Cream

Ingredients
2 cups full-fat coconut milk
1 cup homemade almond milk *
½ cup raw honey
5 large egg yolks **
¼ cup loose leaf earl grey tea
1 tbsp dried culinary grade lavender ***
1 tsp pure vanilla extract

Instructions
Heat coconut and almond milk with the honey over low heat in a saucepan. Make sure it does not boil.
Once milk is hot and honey has been dissolved, remove from heat.
Place the earl grey tea and lavender in a large cotton or paper tea bag and drop it into the milk mixture. Cover saucepan and infuse the milk with tea for 30 minutes (or longer for a much stronger flavor).
Remove tea bag and rewarm the milk over low heat.
At the same time, beat the egg yolks with the vanilla extract and temper it 1 tbsp at a time with the warm milk (until about ¼ cup of milk has been added to the eggs).
Add the rest of the milk to the egg yolk mixture and mix until combined.
Add it back to the pan and heat the mixture over low heat while stirring constantly.
Watch this part carefully to avoid curdling.
Once the mixture has thickened enough to coat the back of a wooden spoon. Remove it from heat and chill for 4-5 hours in the fridge.
Freeze the cooled mixture using an ice cream maker for about 12 minutes. Make sure it does not get too hard.
Place ice cream in a container and freeze for another hour before serving.
This makes a pint of ice cream.

Notes
Homemade almond milk is creamier and has no preservatives compared to the store bought brands.
**Make sure egg yolks are brought to room temperature to avoid curdling.
*** Not all types of dried lavender is edible. Get ones that are used for cooking/baking

147. Blueberry Cream Pie

Ingredients
Crust:
3 cups almonds
½ Teaspoon cinnamon
½ cup honey
2 Tablespoons coconut oil
1 Tablespoon lemon zest
1 Teaspoon almond extract
pinch of sea salt
Filling:
2 Teaspoons kosher plant-based gelatin, dissolved in 2 Tablespoons hot water
⅓ cup freshly squeezed lemon juice
⅓ cup honey
1 can coconut milk, chilled (Native Forest brand is good for this recipe)
4 cups blueberries for serving
Instructions
Place the almonds and cinnamon in a food processor and pulse until your desired texture is reached. I like to leave some bigger pieces for texture. Add the rest of the crust ingredients and pulse until a sticky dough forms. Pat the crust into a pie plate, (use water to keep your hands from sticking to the crust).
For the filling, mix the gelatin and water together. Stir to dissolve and immediately add the lemon juice. If the gelatin gets clumpy, place the mixture over hot water until it melts again. Pour the coconut milk into an electric mixer, add the honey and whip on high until peaks form, about 15 minutes. Add the gelatin mixture to the whipped cream. Pour the filling into the crust. The filling will seem thin, but don't worry it will set up in the refrigerator.
Chill for at least 4 hours until set, and serve with lots of berries!
Notes
Use Grade A maple syrup in place of honey for a completely Vegan version.

148. Gluten Free Dairy Free Coconut

Ingredients
3 cans (14 ounces each) coconut milk, 2 of the 3 refrigerated for at least 24 hours*
3/4 cup (150 g) sugar
1 teaspoon (3 g) unflavored powdered gelatin
3 ounces dairy-free chocolate chips (optional)
1 teaspoon pure vanilla extract (optional)
*You must use full-fat coconut milk. Thai Kitchen brand coconut milk and Whole Foods 365 brand coconut milk both work well consistently for this application.
Directions
In a large, heavy-bottom saucepan, place the entire contents of the 1 room-temperature can of coconut milk and the sugar, and mix to combine well. Cook over medium-high heat, stirring frequently to prevent it from splattering, until it is reduced at least by half and thickened (about 10 minutes). You can also cook the mixture over low heat for about 35 minutes, and stir much less frequently. This is now your sweetened condensed coconut milk. Remove from the heat and set aside to allow to cool completely.
Remove the remaining two cans of coconut milk carefully from the refrigerator, without shaking them at all. The solid should have separated from the liquid while it was chilling, and you don't want to reintegrate them. Remove the lids from the cans, scoop out only the solid white coconut (discarding all of the liquid), and place it in a large bowl. With a hand mixer (or in the bowl of a stand mixer fitted with the whisk attachment), whip the coconut on high speed for about 2 minutes, or until light and fluffy and nearly doubled in volume. Place the whipped coconut cream in the refrigerator to chill for about 10 minutes.
Place the gelatin in a small bowl, and mix well with 2 tablespoons of the sweetened condensed coconut milk from the first step. Allow to sit for 5 minutes while the gelatin dissolves. The mixture will swell. Microwave on 70% power for 20 seconds to liquify the gelatin, and then add the mixture to the rest of the cooled sweetened condensed coconut milk.
Remove the coconut whipped cream from the refrigerator and add the sweetened condensed coconut milk mixture and optional vanilla to it. Whip once more until light and creamy, and well-combined (another 1 to 2 minutes). Fold in optional chocolate chips, and scrape the mixture into a 2 quart freezer-safe container. Cover tightly and freeze until firm (about 6 hours). Serve frozen. If it is at all difficult to scoop, allow to sit in the refrigerator for 15 minutes before scooping and serving.

149. Grain Free Steamed Christmas Puddings – GAPS & Paleo Friendly

Ingredients
150g sultanas
80g dried sour cherries or dried unsweetened cranberries, plus extra for garnish
100g currants
30g activated or raw almonds, roughly chopped
200g kombucha or freshly squeezed orange juice
zest of 1 orange
40g blanched almond meal
20g coconut flour
1/4 tsp nutmeg
1/2 tsp mixed spice
1/4 tsp cinnamon
55g tallow or coconut oil
40g apple, peeled & cored
2 eggs
1/4 tsp fine salt
1/4 tsp bicarb soda

Instructions
Weigh dried fruit and almonds into the Thermo mix bowl, and add kombucha or orange juice.
Cook 6 mins/80C/reverse/speed soft. Remove to a large bowl and set aside to cool.
Place orange zest into clean, dry Thermo mix bowl and chop 20 sec/speed 10.
Add almond meal, coconut flour, spices, salt, soda, apple, eggs and tallow or coconut oil into Thermo mix bowl and mix 5 sec/speed 5. Scrape down sides of bowl.
Add soaked fruit and nuts back to bowl and mix 10 sec/reverse/speed 3.
Scoop mixture into silicone cupcake cups or small ramekins and place into the Varoma dish and tray, with lid on. Cups/ramekins should be about 3/4 full.
Place 500g water into Thermo mix bowl and place Varoma in position. Cook 25 mins/Varoma/speed 2.
Allow puddings to cool, covered, and store in fridge until needed.
Drizzle with Coconut Vanilla Custard, with a dried cranberry or sour cherry on top for decoration.
Notes
I use my Thermo mix to make these puddings - if you don't have a Thermo mix, chop by hand, cook fruit gently on stovetop, and mix in remaining ingredients. Steam in a steamer or use traditional Christmas pudding cooking method.

150. Raw Pineapple Coconut Vegan Cheesecake

Crust:
4 dates, soaked until very soft 1 cup dried organic, unsweetened coconut
Place soften dates and coconut in food processor and process until well blended. Pat into the bottom of an oiled 7 1/2 inch spring form pan.

Filling:
2 1/2 cups young Thai coconut flesh (about 5 young coconuts) 1/4 cup coconut water (from the coconuts) 1/3 cup raw agave nectar or liquid sweetener of choice 1 cup coconut oil, softened 2 cups fresh pineapple chunks, separated

In high-speed blender, pureé the coconut flesh and coconut water together until smooth. Add the agave, coconut oil. You want this to be quite smooth so blend away until it is. Add 1 cup of the pineapple chunks. Blend until incorporated. Pulse the remaining pineapple chunks in the food processor until well chopped. Drain. Stir the pineapple into the coconut mixture, pour over crust and let set up in the refrigerator for 4 hours. Move to freezer and leave until firm.

151. Grain-free Italian Lemon Almond Cake

Ingredients

320 grams (this is about 3 cups + 3 tablespoons) almond flour (not almond meal) or blanched almonds, ground into almond flour
200 grams (1 cup + 3 tablespoons) white chocolate, chopped
2 tablespoons whipping cream or milk (I used 1.5% milk)
180 grams (3/4 cup + 1 tablespoon) unsalted butter, softened
130 grams (about 2/3 cup) granulated sugar or coconut sugar1
zest of 4 lemons, about 2 tablespoons
4 large eggs, separated
1 teaspoon lemon extract
40 grams (about 2 tablespoons) of limoncello or lemon juice
powdered sugar as garnish, optional

Directions

Preheat your oven to 350°F / 176°C and grease a 10" / 26cm pan or line it with parchment paper. If using blanched almonds instead of almond flour, process them in the food processor until they're pretty finely ground. If you grind them too much, they'll release oil and become almond butter.
Combine the white chocolate and milk / cream in a microwave safe bowl.
Heat in 30 second increments and stir after every 30 seconds. Set aside to cool while you prepare the rest. Beat the butter with 100 grams of sugar and beat until fluffy.
Add the lemon zest, egg yolks and lemon extract and beat until well combined. Then add the almond flour / ground almonds and the melted chocolate. Add the limoncello / lemon juice and beat until combined.
In a separate bowl with spotlessly clean beaters, beat the egg whites until soft peaks form. Gradually add the remaining 30 grams of sugar to the egg white mixture. Fold the egg whites into the almond batter until well combined. Spoon the batter into the greased pan and bake for 40 - 45 minutes. If making half the cake, use a 7" / 18cm pan and bake for 30 minutes. The cake will puff up in the oven, but when cooling, it'll fall back down.
Let it cool completely in the pan and then invert the cake onto a plate, and then flip that back into the pan or onto another plate (so that it's not upside down). Sprinkle on some powdered sugar if desired, but only before serving.
Notes

If using coconut sugar, blend in a coffee grinder first so that it's basically like powdered coconut sugar. I'd be worried about how well non-grinded coconut sugar would do with the egg whites. I'm guessing not well. And please note the above comment about how using coconut sugar turns the cake the brown! It's just not possible to make a bright yellow cake with this dark sugar. Also, this recipe originally used 200 grams of sugar. I used 200 grams in the first cake and only 130 in the second and didn't notice much of a difference, but I'm used to not using so much sugar. Feel free to use up to 200 grams.

152. Cheeky Cherry Crisp

Ingredients:
3 cups cherries, pitted and sliced
2 tsp almond extract
1/3 cup unsweetened coconut milk
A few drops stevia to taste

For the topping:
1/4 cup hemp seeds
1/4 cup almond flour
1/4 cup coconut flour
2 Tbl coconut oil
1 Tbl water
1 tsp cinnamon
pinch of low sodium salt

Instructions:
In a medium bowl, combine the cherries, almond extract, coconut milk and sweetener if using. Make sure there are no pits!
In another bowl combine all of the topping ingredients and mix well until crumbly.
Pour the cherry filling into one large, 4 medium, or 8 small greased ramekins or oven proof dishes.
Top with the crumble mixture and bake for 20 minutes in a preheated 375 degree (F) oven. Remove from the oven and let cool before serving. Yum!

153. Stunning Key Lime Pie

Ingredients:
Filling:
6 avocados
3-4 drops stevia
1 cup coconut oil
2/3 cup lime juice

Crust :
1 1/2 cups almond flour/meal
2 TBSP almond butter
3-4 drops stevia
1/4 cup unsweetened coconut, shredded
1/4 cup coconut flour

Instructions:
Place all crust ingredients in food processor and pulse until grainy. It should stick together when you press on it, but not form a ball by itself. If it does, add more almond flour.
Dump blended ingredients into spring form pan and press down to form crust.
Wipe out food processor and place all filling ingredients within. Blend for several minutes (4-5) until completely smooth. Pour over crust and smooth out.
Place pie in freezer for 1-2 hours. Serve chilled.

154. Delectable Cocoa-Nut Apples

Ingredients:
1 ½ cups coconut flakes
2 tablespoons cacao powder
1 tablespoon cacao nibs
1 ½ teaspoons cinnamon
1/8 teaspoon nutmeg
3-4 drops stevia
1 organic green apple
2 tablespoons heated coconut oil
A half tablespoon of water if consistency is too dry

Instructions:
In a medium sized mixing bowl add coconut flakes, cacao powder, cacao nibs, cinnamon, nutmeg and coconut oil. Stir well, for 2-3 minutes, Clean and dry the apple. Thinly slice the apple starting from the outside and working your way toward the center. Repeat on the other side. Then lay the apple flat on one of the cut sides and chop thin slices of the remaining sides of the apple core
Transfer the sliced apple to a serving tray.
Pour the cocoa-nut mixture on top of each apple.
Now you can serve them right away or let them sit for an hour or longer to let the coconut flake mixture soften, totally up to you.

155. Outstanding Hazelnut Banana

Ingredients:
1 banana, sliced
1 tablespoon hazelnut butter
Cinnamon
Olive oil or coconut oil

Instructions:
Lightly drizzle oil in a skillet over medium heat.
Arrange banana slices in pan and cook for 1-2 minutes on each side.
Remove pan from heat and place bits of hazelnut butter over banana.
Allow to cool and sprinkle with cinnamon.

156. Cookies with Dark Chocolate

Ingredients:
2.5 cups unsweetened dark chocolate, in 1 oz chunks
3 large eggs
1/3 C coconut oil
3/4 drops stevia
1 T vanilla
3/4-1 C almond flour(sunflower seed flour for nut-free)
1/4 C organic cocoa powder
1/4 teaspoon low sodium salt
1/4 teaspoon baking powder
coarse low sodium sea salt or pink low sodium salt for sprinkling

Instructions:
Melt chocolate together into a smooth consistency (double boiler or microwave in blasts of 30-60 seconds), stirring constantly and making sure that one does not over cook or seize before they both come together.
Sift dry ingredients and set aside. Combine wet ingredients, except chocolate, by whisking until combined.
Temper in melted chocolate by adding in about 1/4 C and whisking. Then add another 1/4 C of the warm chocolate and whisk again. Then add the remaining melted chocolate to the remaining wet batter.
Slowly add in the dry ingredients, stirring on low until just incorporated together - final batter will be smooth and plyable.
If you used 3/4 C flour you'll want to set your dough aside to chill for a little while, only 10 minutes or so. This will allow the chocolate to cool a bit and make the dough more plyable. If you used 1 C flour, the dough should be firm enough to shape into balls right away.
Form tablespoon sized balls, sprinkle with low sodium salt then press semi-flat onto a parchment-lined baking sheet. Bake at 350 degrees for 9 minutes, or until the center of the cookie begins to firm - will further harden as it rests.

157. Lemon Almond Delight

Ingredients:
6 Tbl coconut oil
2 cups almond flour
3-4 drops stevia
1 tsp freshly grated lemon zest

Instructions:
Melt the butter in the microwave or a small saucepan. Add the almond flour, stevia, and lemon zest, stirring until fully combined.
To make a tart or pie crust:
No need to pre-chill, just press dough into tart or pie tins. Bake in a preheated oven at 350 degrees (F) for 15 mins until firm and golden brown.
To make the cookies:
Form dough (it will be crumbly, this is normal) into a cylinder and wrap tightly with plastic wrap to compress. Chill in freezer for 30 minutes or until firm, or in the refrigerator for 2 hours. With a sharp knife, slice into 1/2 inch thick cookies (if they crumble apart your dough isn't cold enough). Bake in a preheated oven @ 350 degrees (F) on a greased or parchment lined cookie sheet for 15 minutes, or until firm and golden brown. Allow to cool before removing.

158. Ginger Vanilla Extravaganza

Ingredients:
3-4 drops stevia
3 Tbsp Organic Coconut Oil
2.5 cup Blanched Almond Flour
1/2 tsp low sodium Salt
1/2 tsp Baking Soda
1/2 tsp ground Cloves
1/2 tsp ground Cinnamon
1/2 tsp ground Nutmeg
1/2 tsp ground Ginger
More stevia to taste – administer the drops slowly

Instructions:
Preheat oven to 350 degrees.
In a large mixing bowl, combine blanched almond flour, low sodium salt, baking soda, cloves, cinnamon, nutmeg, ginger, and stevia. Stir ingredients with a wooden spoon to combine.
In a small sauce pan, bring molasses to a boil over medium heat.
Add coconut oil to the sauce pan, and stir until combined with the molasses.
Remove sauce pan from heat and pour into the dry ingredients.
Mix batter with a wooden spoon until you have formed a dark golden cookie dough, and all the dry ingredients are combined with the molasses and coconut oil.
Place a sheet of parchment paper onto a flat cooking surface, and dust parchment with arrowroot flour.
Form dough into a ball, and place on the parchment paper. Lightly press dough down to flatten, and sprinkle with a small amount of arrowroot flour. Place another sheet of parchment paper on top of the dough, and roll into a thin sheet with a rolling pin (about 1/4 inch thick).
Sprinkle almond flour on a small plate, and place cookie cutters into the arrowroot to coat the bottom for cutting. This will keep the cookie dough from sticking to the batter for an easy release after cutting.
Once you have made cuts throughout the entire sheet of cookie dough, carefully peel away the excess dough, and lightly transfer the cut out cookies to a parchment lined baking sheet. Form dough into another ball, and roll out again to repeat until all the dough is used.
Bake gingerbread people at 350 degrees for 10 minutes. Remove from oven and cool on a cookie rack before frosting.

159. Cute Cupcakes Recipe

Ingredients:
2/3 Cup coconut flour
1/4 Cup almond flour
1/2 tsp cinnamon
1 tsp baking powder
1/2 tsp low sodium salt
6 eggs
2 egg whites
304 drops stevia
1 Tbsp vanilla
1/2 Cup coconut milk (canned)

Buttercream Frosting Recipe
1 1/4 Cup Grass-fed Butter softened (20 T. or 2 ¼ sticks)
3-4 drops stevia
1/2 tsp cinnamon
2 1/2 Tbsp coconut flour
5 Tbsp coconut cream (the thick coconut cream skimmed off the top of canned coconut milk)
1/4 tsp cinnamon

Instructions:
Preheat the oven to 350 degrees.
Line 2 muffin tins with a total of 16 cupcake liners.
Place the coconut flour, almond flour, cinnamon, baking powder, and low sodium salt in a small bowl and mix together with a whisk.
In another bowl, combine the eggs, egg whites, stevia, vanilla, and coconut milk, beating together well with a whisk.
Add the dry ingredients to the wet ingredients, whisking until well combined.
Add the melted butter to the batter and mix in well.
Let the batter sit for 5 minutes to allow the coconut flour time to absorb the liquids.
Divide batter evenly between cupcake liners and bake for 20-22 minutes, or until tops of cake are firm to the touch and spring back.
Remove and cool completely on a wire rack.

Buttercream Frosting Instructions
Place the butter, stevia, cinnamon, and coconut flour in a bowl and beat with a mixer until well combined.
Beat in the coconut cream, 1 t. at a time, until fully incorporated.
Mixture should be thick and glossy.
Scoop into a piping back and pipe on top of cooled cupcakes.
Mix more stevia and ¼ t. cinnamon together and sprinkle desired amount on top of cupcakes.

Paleo Diet Recipes 365 Days of Paleo and Coconut Recipes by Mercedes Del Rey

160. Strawberry Chessecake Delight

Ingredients:
1 cup almonds course ground
1 heaping cup soaked raw cashews (soaked overnight or at least 4 hours)
1/2 cup peeled and diced zucchini
1/4 cup coconut oil, melted
2 tablespoons canned coconut milk, full fat, room temperature
4-5 drops stevia
1/2 tablespoon vanilla extract
1/8 teaspoon low sodium salt
juice of one and a half lemons, separated
1 cup fresh organic strawberries, hulled and diced

Instructions:
Divide the cup of almond crumbs into the bottom of 4 (8-ounce) wide mouth mason jars and set them aside.
In a high-powered blender, process the raw cashews until they are blended. Add the zucchini, coconut oil, coconut milk, stevia, vanilla extract, low sodium salt, and the juice of one lemon. For the lemon juice go by taste as not to overdo it with lemon flavor. I started by juicing half of the lemon, mixing and tasting, and adding the rest. Add lemon juice as needed to your preference. Then blend again until a super smooth and creamy batter is formed.
Pour the cheesecake batter evenly into the 4 (8-ounce) wide mouth mason jars leaving some room for the strawberry sauce. Place them in the freezer and allow them to set for at least an hour or longer. While the cheesecake is setting go ahead and make your strawberry sauce.
In a heavy bottomed sauce pot over medium-high heat, add the juice of half a lemon, the strawberries, and honey. Mash the strawberries together until they are combined with the rest of the ingredients. Let the mixture boil and reduce, stirring intermittently, for about 10-12 minutes or so. Once the mixture has reduced and thickened remove from heat and set aside.
When your cheesecake is ready, remove mason jars from the freezer, let thaw for about 15 minutes before serving. Top with strawberry sauce. Garnish with fresh strawberry slices and a sprinkle of almond crumbs. Enjoy!

161. Creative Cardamom Cupcakes

Ingredients:
1/2 cup coconut flour
6 eggs, at room temperature (that's important)
3-4 drops. stevia
6 Tbs. coconut oil or butter
2 Tbs. coconut milk, room temp. (this one doesn't have any icky additives or BPA)
1 tsp. vanilla extract
1/2 tsp. ground cardamom
1/4 tsp. baking soda
1/2 tsp. apple cider vinegar

Instructions:
Preheat the oven to 350 degrees and prepare a muffin tin with 8 liners (I like unbleached parchment paper baking cups).
Combine the coconut flour and eggs until smooth. Add the remaining ingredients and stir well.
Divide evenly between the muffin tins. Bake until golden and a toothpick comes out clean, about 20 minutes.
Cool completely and frost with the lemon mousse.
Makes 8 cupcakes. Feel free to double the recipe if you want more cupcakes! These last in an airtight container for a few days at room temperature. They also freeze really well!

162. Apple, almond & blackberry Bonanza

Ingredients:
Filling:
3 sweet apples
100 g blackberries, frozen are fine
3-4 drops stevia
1 knob of coconut oil
1/2 tsp cinnamon
1/4 tsp cardamom
1/8 tsp cloves/all spice
1/8 tsp ground ginger

Batter:
3/4 cup ground almonds (100 g)
2 Tbsp stevia
1/2 tsp ground vanilla
1/2 tsp baking powder
a pinch of low sodium salt
1 Tbsp melted coconut oil or butter
1 egg, whisked
Around 1/5 cup full fat coconut milk(50 ml)

Instructions:
Preheat oven to 200 °C/ 400 °F. Cut apples on bite-sized chunks. You need to use an oven proof skillet* about 20 cm i diameter. Melt coconut oil and stevia on high heat and add the apples and spices.
Sauté for 5 min until the apples are caramelized and slightly tender.
Meanwhile make the batter. Mix almond flour with vanilla, stevia, baking powder and low sodium salt. Stir in the egg, coconut oil and coconut milk.
Place the blackberries among the apples in the skillet. Pour the batter on top if the fruit until it covers the surface. It is okay if there is small cracks where the fruit can release some moist.
Bake in the oven for 15-20 min. depending on your oven. The cake should be golden brown on the entire surface and the batter just set.
Serve the cake while it is still a little warm with a dollop of yoghurt, whipped cream or splash of coconut milk – and maybe a few fresh black berries on top.. Enjoy.

163. Almond Happiness Bars

Ingredients:
First Layer:
3/4 cup raw almond butter (I make my own from this recipe: Almond Butter)
1/4 cup coconut oil, melted
1/3 cup cacao powder
3-4 drops stevia
1/4 teaspoon vanilla bean paste
pinch low sodium salt

Second Layer:
2 cups of dried, unsweetened, raw coconut
2/3 cup coconut butter, softened
3-4 drops stevia
1-2 teaspoons organic almond flavoring (not raw)

Third Layer:
1/3 cup almonds, coarsely chopped

Ganache:
1/2 cup cacao powder
3-4 drops stevia
1/4 cup coconut oil, melted

Instructions:
First Layer:
Whisk all ingredients together and pour into oiled, parchment lined 8 x 8-inch glass pan. Set in refrigerator aside making topping. The bottom layer should be set up (but not completely hard) before adding the next layer.

Second Layer:
Place coconut in medium bowl.
Whisk coconut butter (not the same as coconut oil), agave and almond flavor. Pour over coconut and mix well.
Pat over first layer, top with chopped almonds and ganache.
Refrigerate to set.

Ganache:
Whisk all ingredients together.

164. Sexy Coconut Crack Bars

Ingredients:
1 cup unsweetened shredded coconut (80g)
1/4 cup water and 2-3 drops stevia
2 tbsp virgin coconut oil (For all substitutions in this recipe, see nutrition link below)
1/2 tsp pure vanilla extract
1/8 tsp low sodium salt
Instructions:
Combine all ingredients in a food processor....and fridge for an hour before trying to cut. (Or freeze for 15 minutes.) Can be stored in the fridge or freezer, for at least a few weeks.

165. Lemonny Lemon Delights

Ingredients:
Crust:
1 cup almond flour
1/4 cup almond butter
Stevia to taste
1 tbsp coconut butter
1 tsp vanilla
1/2 tsp baking powder
1/4 tsp low sodium salt
Filling:
3 eggs
A few drops Stevia to taste
1/4 cup lemon juice
2 1/2 tbsp coconut flour
1 tbsp lemon zest, finely grated
Pinch of low sodium salt
Instructions:
Preheat oven to 350.
Coat 9×9 baking dish with coconut oil or butter.
Combine all crust ingredients in food processor until a "crumble" forms.
Press crust evenly into the bottom of pan.
Using a fork, prick a few holes into crust.
Bake for 10 minutes.
While crust is baking, combine all filling ingredients in a food processor until well incorporated.
When done, remove crust from oven and pour filling evenly over top.
Continue to bake for 15-20 minutes, or until filling is set, but still has a little jiggle.
Cool completely on wire rack. (You can also chill in the fridge if desired, to further set the filling).

166. Macadamia Pineapple Bonanza

Ingredients:
Crust:
½ cup almond flour
4 tablespoons raw cacao powder
⅓ cup macadamia nuts
½ teaspoon vanilla extract
Stevia to taste
1½ teaspoons coconut oil, melted

Filling:
2 eggs
1 cup fresh pineapple, chopped
1⅓ cup shredded coconut, unsweetened
1 tablespoon fresh lime juice
1 tablespoon vanilla extract
Stevia to taste
½ cup almond flour
pinch of low sodium salt

Instructions:
Crust:
In a large bowl, mix the almond flour and cacao powder.
Chop the macadamia nuts in a food processor and add it to the bowl.
Add vanilla extract and coconut oil to the dry mixture and using your hands, mix to combine ingredients.
Spread the mixture evenly on the bottom of an 8x8-inch pan lined with parchment paper. Be sure to use one large piece of paper covering the entire pan that overlaps on all four sides.

Filing:
In a large bowl beat the 2 eggs
Mix in the pineapple, 1 cup of shredded coconut (reserve the remaining ⅓ cup for the top), lime juice, vanilla and stevia.
Gently mix in the almond flour and low sodium salt with rubber spatula.
Pour mixture over the crust and sprinkle top with remaining shredded coconut.
Bake at 350°F for approximately 20 minutes or until the top starts to brown and the pineapple/coconut layer is firm.
Set pan on a wire rack and allow it to cool before cutting into squares. Store in the refrigerator.

167. Pretty Pumpkin Delights

Ingredients:
For Crust:
1 cup hazelnuts (preferably soaked and dehydrated for better digestion)
1/2 cup raw pumpkin seeds (preferably soaked and dehydrated for better digestion)
1 TBS coconut oil
2 pinches of low sodium salt
Stevia to taste

For Filling:
1 cup cooked pumpkin puree
1/2 cup coconut
2 TBS coconut oil
Stevia to taste
1/2 tsp vanilla extract
1/4 tsp cinnamon powder
1/4 tsp ginger powder
1/8 tsp allspice
1/8 tsp clove powder

For Chocolate Drizzle:
2 TBS coconut butter
2 TBS coconut oil
2 TBS raw cacao (or unsweetened cocoa)
Stevia to taste
a pinch or 2 of low sodium salt

Instructions:
To Make the crust: Line mini muffin tins with unbleached mini paper liners. Process all crust ingredients in a food processor until well combined and resembles a coarse flour. Spoon 1 and 1/2 tsp of mixture into each of the 24 mini cups. Use your thumb to press down mixture firmly to create a solid bottom layer for these cute little yummies. Place in freezer to harden.
To make filling: Melt coconut butter and coconut oil in a double boiler. Remove from heat and add rest of filling ingredients. Go ahead and mix it up real good here until creamy smooth. Remove crusts from freezer and spoon about 3/4 TBS of filling over your prepared crusts. Return to freezer to harden, at least 2 hours.
To make chocolate drizzle: Once mini bites have hardened, gently melt coconut butter and coconut oil in a double boiler. Remove from heat and add rest of drizzle ingredients. Allow to cool slightly to thicken. Pour into small plastic bag, cut a TINY hole in the corner, and drizzle over treats in any fashion that you want.
Now it's time to enjoy these amazing delights. Store leftovers in freezer as they are best cold. (That is, if there are any leftovers. Ours got dusted off in one day.)

168. Sexy Dessert Pan

Ingredients:
Crust:
1 1/2 cups pecans
3/4 cup dates
4 tbsp coconut oil

Second Layer:
2/3 cup cashew butter
1/3 cup palm shortening
2 tsp apple cider vinegar
1/2 tsp lemon juice
Pinch low sodium salt

Third Layer:
1 cup coconut flour
1 cup coconut milk
Stevia to taste
1 tsp vanilla extract

Fourth Layer:
1/2 cup coconut milk
1/2 cup coconut butter
1/2 cup cacao powder
2 tbsp honey

Fifth Layer:
1/2 cup coconut butter
1/4 cup coconut milk
Stevia to taste

Sixth Layer:
Grated dark sugar free chocolate, at least 80% cacao

Instructions:
To make the crust, roughly chop the pecans then pit and chop the dates. Load both into a food processor and pulse until ground but still crumbly. Transfer to a bowl and work in the coconut oil, then press the sticky mixture into a single smooth layer at the bottom of a square 8x8 cake pan.
Transfer to the refrigerator to chill while you begin the second layer. To make the second layer, combine its ingredients very well in a medium mixing bowl. Spoon over the chilled crust, smoothing as much as possible with the back of a spoon. Place the pan back in the fridge.
To make the third layer, mix its ingredients together in a mixing bowl and then spoon over the chilled, hardened second layer. Smooth as much as possible, then chill.
Add the fourth layer by combining its ingredients and then layering it into the pan in the same way as the previous layers.

For the fifth layer, mix the coconut shortening, coconut milk and stevia with a hand mixer until very smooth and spoon over the chilled fourth layer.

Before placing the pan back into the refrigerator after adding the fifth layer, grate very dark chocolate over the top to the depth of your preference. Chill the pan for an additional half hour or more, then slice with a sharp knife and serve.

Notes:
The layers may seem fiddly but the technique is so simple once you're in the thick of it: just mix the ingredients, spoon into the pan and chill!

169. Peachy Creamy Peaches

Ingredients:
3 medium ripe peaches, cut in half with pit removed
1 tsp vanilla
1 can coconut milk, refrigerated
1/4 cup chopped walnuts
Cinnamon (to taste)

Instructions:
Place peaches on the grill with the cut side down first. Grill on medium-low heat until soft, about 3-5 minutes on each side. Scoop cream off the top of the can of chilled coconut milk. Whip together coconut cream and vanilla with handheld mixer. Drizzle over each peach. Top with cinnamon and chopped walnuts to garnish.

170. Creamy Berrie Pie

Ingredients:
Crust:
3 cups almonds
½ Teaspoon cinnamon
½ cup honey
2 Tablespoons coconut oil
1 Tablespoon lemon zest
1 Teaspoon almond extract
pinch of low sodium salt
Filling:
2 Teaspoons plant-based gelatin, dissolved in 2 Tablespoons hot water
⅓ cup freshly squeezed lemon juice
Stevia to taste
1 can coconut milk, chilled
4 cups blueberries for serving
Instructions:
Place the almonds and cinnamon in a food processor and pulse until your desired texture is reached. I like to leave some bigger pieces for texture. Add the rest of the crust ingredients and pulse until a sticky dough forms. Pat the crust into a pie plate, (use water to keep your hands from sticking to the crust).
For the filling, mix the gelatin and water together. Stir to dissolve and immediately add the lemon juice. If the gelatin gets clumpy, place the mixture over hot water until it melts again. Pour the coconut milk into an electric mixer, add the stevia and whip on high until peaks form, about 15 minutes. Add the gelatin mixture to the whipped cream. Pour the filling into the crust. The filling will seem thin, but don't worry it will set up in the refrigerator.
Chill for at least 4 hours until set, and serve with lots of berries!

171. Choco - Coconut Berry Ice

Ingredients:
Follow recipe of berry ice cream and almond delight for the ice cream only
4 ounces sugar free dark chocolate - 75% cacao content
¼ cup coconut milk
2 cups fresh berries (I used raspberries)

Instructions:
Make the Homemade Coconut Ice Cream,

While the ice cream is freezing in the machine, break the chocolate into pieces and place in a small saucepan.

Add the coconut milk and melt the two together, stirring over low heat.

When the chocolate mixture is completely smooth, pour the chocolate over the ice cream and stir to create 'ripples'. If your ice cream if thoroughly frozen, soften in the fridge for 20 minutes before stirring in the chocolate.

Serve immediately with the fresh berries, or freeze for an additional 3-4 hours for a firmer texture.

172. Cheeky Cherry Ice

Ingredients:
14oz. cans 365 Coconut Milk (Full Fat)
Stevia to taste
1 ½ tsp. vanilla extract
2 cups fresh cherries, pitted and diced

Instructions:
In a large bowl, combine coconut milk, stevia and vanilla and stir well.
Chill for 1-2 hours.
Transfer to ice-cream maker and process according to manufacturer directions.
Add diced cherries to the mixture during the last 5-10 minutes of processing.

173. Creamy Caramely Ice Cream

Ingredients:
Delicious Instant Caramel Topping:
2 heaped tablespoons of hulled tahini
Stevia to taste
2 tablespoons of coconut milk
1/2 teaspoon of vanilla

Delicious Instant Ice Cream:
4 frozen bananas, chopped
4 tablespoons coconut milk
1 teaspoon of vanilla

Instructions:
Spoon the tahini and stevia into a cup and stir with a fork to combine. Mix in the coconut milk and vanilla. Refrain from eating it while you make your ice cream.
Place the ingredients into food processor or blender, blend until the mixture is an ice cream consistency.
Spoon the ice cream into bowls, drizzle generously with the caramel topping, sprinkle with low sodium salt if you desire. Enjoy!

174. Berry Ice Cream and Almond Delight

Ingredients:
For the Ice Cream:
1 can full fat coconut milk
Stevia to taste
2 tbsp vanilla
1 cup fresh strawberries, cut into fourths

For the crisp:
1/3 cup almond flour
3 tbsp sunflower seed butter (or almond butter)
1/2 tsp vanilla
1 tbsp honey
low sodium salt to taste

Instructions:
For the ice cream:
Combine coconut milk and vanilla together in a small saucepan over medium heat and stir until ingredients are well combined (just a few minutes).
Transfer milk mixture to a small bowl and place in the freezer for two hours.
Next, add strawberries to a small saucepan and bring to a low boil.
Turn heat to medium-low and allow to cook until they start breaking down into a sauce-like mixture, leaving small chunks.
Place strawberries in refrigerator while the ice cream hardens.
For the crisp:
Combine all ingredients and mix until you get a "crumble' consistency.
Place crisp in refrigerator until ready to use.
After two hours, place milk mixture into your ice cream maker along with the strawberries and use as directed.
When ice cream is ready, scoop and serve with crisp sprinkled on top.

175. Eastern Spice Delights

Ingredients:
1 3/4 cups + 4 tbsp almond meal
1/8 tsp low sodium salt
3/4 tsp ground ginger
3/4 tsp cinnamon
1/4 tsp ground cloves
1/4 tsp cardamom
1/8 tsp nutmeg
1/2 cup coconut oil (in solid form)
Stevia to taste
1 tsp vanilla extract
Instructions:
Preheat oven to 350F.
Combine all the dry ingredients in a large bowl. In a small bowl, mix together the oil, maple syrup, and vanilla until completely blended. Pour the wet ingredients over the dry ingredients and mix well.
Drop the cookie dough on a cookie sheet. It will spread a bit as it cooks (and thus flatten), but not an awful lot.
Bake for 10-12 minutes. These cookies will not look golden when they're done. Makes two dozens.

176. Absolute Almond Bites

Ingredients:
1 1/2 cups almond flour
1/4 teaspoon low sodium salt
1/4 teaspoon baking soda (gluten-free, if necessary)
1/8 teaspoon cinnamon
2 tablespoons melted coconut oil
Stevia to taste
1 1/4 teaspoon vanilla extract
1/4 teaspoon almond extract or almond flavoring
12 to 15 whole almonds; sprouted or soaked and dehydrated

Instructions:
Preheat oven to 325°F. Line a baking sheet with parchment paper.
In a medium bowl combine almond flour, low sodium salt, baking soda, and cinnamon. Mix well, breaking up any lumps.
In a small bowl, place coconut oil, vanilla, almond extract or flavoring. Whisk until well combined.
Add wet ingredients to dry ingredients and stir until combined...add stevia
Roll level-tablespoon-sized (using a measuring spoon) portions of dough into balls and place on baking sheet. Flatten slightly with the heel of your hand and press one almond into the center of each cookie.
Bake 15 to 17 minutes or until light golden brown. Allow to cool on baking sheet for a few minutes before transferring to cooling rack.
Store in an airtight container. Can be frozen.

177. Choco Coco Cookies

Ingredients:
Stevia powder – 1 teaspoon
1 cup coconut flour
½ cup coconut oil
½ cup coconut milk, (from the can)
2 Teaspoons vanilla extract
¼ Teaspoon low sodium salt
2½ cups finely shredded coconut
1 cup big flake coconut
⅔ cup dark sugar free chocolate chunks or chocolate chips (I used 80% dark chocolate)
Optional: ½ cup almond or cashew butter
Instructions:
In a large saucepan, combine the, coconut oil, and coconut milk. Bring the mixture to a boil, and boil for 2-3 minutes.
Remove from the heat and add the vanilla, low sodium salt, and coconut flour and coconut. Stir to combine. If you're using the almond or cashew butter, mix it in thoroughly. Finally, add the chocolate chunks and combine, stirring as little as possible to keep the chunks intact.
Portion the cookie on a parchment lined baking sheet and let cool. This version of no-bakes takes a full 3-4 hours to fully set up, but you don't have to wait that long because they're really good warm and gooey.

178. Chococups

Ingredients:
4 eggs
Stevia to taste
1/3 cup coconut flour
1/4 cup cacao powder
1/2 teaspoon baking soda
1/4 cup coconut oil (melted in microwave)
1/4 cup cacao butter (melted in microwave)
For topping:
1 can coconut cream (chilled in fridge overnight)
Cacao nibs to decorate.
Instructions:
Heat oven to 170 degrees Celsius (338F)
Grease 10 muffin pans with coconut oil.
Beat eggs with electric beaters.
Add coconut flour, baking soda and cacao powder.
Beat well and add stevia
Add melted coconut oil, cacao butter and mix.
Spoon mixture into 10 greased muffin pans.
Bake for 12-15 minutes until risen and top springs back.
Cool in pans.
Beat the solid coconut cream with electric beaters until creamy. Add honey to taste if you wish.
Pipe coconut cream onto top of cakes.

179. Choco – Almond Delights

Ingredients:
1 c. toasted hazelnuts
1 c. raw almonds
2/3 c. raw almond butter
5 Tbs. raw cacao powder (or unsweetened cocoa powder)
1/2 tsp. vanilla extract
1/4 c. unsweetened, shredded coconut

Instructions:
Combine all the ingredients, except for the coconut, in the food processor. Whir until smooth. This will take a few minutes and may require scraping down the sides of the bowl one or more times.

Line a mini muffin tin with plastic wrap. Spoon dollops of the sweet mixture into the lined tin cups and form into "mounds." Freeze until well formed. Remove mounds from plastic and tin and flip for presentation. Sprinkle with shredded coconut.

180. Fetching Fudge

Ingredients:
1 cup coconut butter
1/4 cup coconut oil
1/4 cup cocoa
1/4 cup cocoa powder + 1 Tbsp
Stevia to taste
1 tsp vanilla

Instructions:
In the pot, gently melt the cocoa butter on low (number 2)
When it is half melted add the butter, the coconut oil and the coconut spread and gently mix with the whisk as it melts
Add vanilla, and stevia and whisk in well
Add the cocoa powder and whisk in well
Be sure to take the pot off the heat when the fat is melted and keep whisking until it is smooth and all the lumps are out — you don't want to overheat this
Pour into the 8 x 8 pan that is lined with parchment paper
Refrigerate for 1 – 2 hours
When solid, pull the parchment paper out of the pan, put the block of fudge on a flat surface and cut into small squares
Enjoy! This will melt rather quickly — but it won't last long!

181. Nut Butter Truffles

Ingredients:
5 tablespoons sunflower seed butter
1 tablespoon coconut oil
2 teaspoons vanilla extract
¾ cup almond flour
1 tablespoon flaxseed meal
pinch of low sodium salt
¼ cup sugar free dark chocolate chips
1 tablespoon cacao butter
chopped almonds (optional)

Instructions:
Add sunflower seed butter, coconut oil, vanilla, almond flour, flaxseed meal and low sodium salt to a large bowl. Please note that you may find a thin layer of oil in the sunflower seed butter jar that separates from the butter and rises to the top. Be sure to mix oil and butter together before scooping into bowl.
Using your hands mix until all ingredients are incorporated (I like using gloves when mixing so the oils from my skin do not get into the mixture)
Roll the dough into 1-inch balls and place them on a sheet of parchment paper and refrigerate for 30 minutes (using 2 teaspoons for each truffle will yield about 14 truffles)
Melt the chocolate chips in a double boiler along with the cacao butter
Dip each truffle in the melted chocolate, one at the time, and place them back on the pan with parchment paper
Top with chopped almonds and refrigerate until the chocolate is firm

182. Extra Dark Choco Delight

Ingredients:
1 egg
½ very ripe avocado
¼ cup full fat canned coconut milk
2 tbsp cacao powder
1 tbsp carob powder
pinch low sodium salt
pinch cinnamon
1 scoop vanilla flavored hemp protein powder
10g raw hazelnuts
2 tbsp unsweetened shredded coconut

Instructions:
Add the egg, avocado and coconut milk to a small food processor and process until very smooth and process until very smooth and creamy.
Add cacao powder, carob powder, low sodium salt, cinnamon and protein powder and process again until well combined and creamy.
Add hazelnuts and shredded coconut and give a few extra spins until the hazelnuts are reduced to tiny little pieces.
Serve immediately or refrigerate until ready to serve.
Garnish with a little dollop of coconut cream and cacao nibs or shredded coconut and crushed hazelnuts.
This will keep in the refrigerator for a few days in an airtight container.

183. Chestnut- Cacao Cake

Ingredients:
100g (1 cup + 1 heaping tablespoon) chestnut flour
50g (1/2 cup) ground almonds (almond flour)
3 eggs, separate
1/2 teaspoon cream of tartar
35g (1/2 cup) raw cacao powder
Stevia to taste
3/4 cup coconut milk
1/2 teaspoon baking soda
Crushed chesnuts

Instructions:
Preheat oven to 180C fan (350F).
Grease a pie/tart pan.
In a clean mixing bowl, beat the egg whites and cream of tartar until stiff peaks form. Set aside.
In another mixing bowl, cream the egg yolks, chestnut flour, ground almonds, stevia, raw cacao, baking soda and coconut milk.
Fold in the egg whites and blend until the white is no longer showing.
Pour into the pie/tart mold.
Sprinkle with crushed chestnuts, if desired.
Bake for 35-40 minutes on the middle rack.

184. Apple Cinnamon Walnut Bonanza

Ingredients:
For the cake:
1 cup almond flour
2 tablespoons coconut flour
Stevia to taste
1 tablespoon cinnamon
1 teaspoon baking soda
1/4 teaspoon low sodium salt
1 tablespoon coconut butter, plus more for greasing the pan
2 eggs
1/2 cup cream from a can of refrigerated coconut milk
1 teaspoon vanilla
1 cup grated apple (about 1 large apple)

For the topping:
1 1/2 cups walnuts (or pecans, if you prefer)
1/2 cup almond flour
4 tablespoons melted coconut butter
Stevia to taste
1 tablespoon cinnamonpinch low sodium salt

Instructions:
Preheat your oven to 350° and grease a 8 x 8 baking dish.
Make the topping: pulse the walnuts in a food processor 10-12 times or until they are course crumbs. Add the remaining ingredients and pulse 2-3 more times until combined. Set aside.
Wipe out and dry the bowl of your food processor and add your dry cake ingredients. (almond flour through low sodium salt) Pulse a few times to mix.
Cut the tablespoon of butter into smaller chunks and add it to the dry ingredients. Pulse 8-10 times or until it's cut in to the dry ingredients, similar to if you were making a pie crust.
In a small bowl, mix your wet cake ingredients (eggs through vanilla) and whisk until well combined. Stir in grated apple.
Add to the food processor and mix until combined. Scrape down the sides once or twice to make sure it's well mixed.
Pour into the prepared baking dish and sprinkle the topping over, as evenly as you can.
Bake for 30-35 minutes, or until a toothpick inserted into the center comes out clean.
Allow to cool, and enjoy!

Paleo Diet Recipes 365 Days of Paleo and Coconut Recipes by Mercedes Del Rey

185. Choco Triple Delight

Ingredients:
Cake:
1 cup almond flour (or 3 oz ground raw pumpkin seeds for nut-free version)
3 tbsp Raw Cacao Powder
1 tbsp coconut flour
1 tsp baking powder
1/2 tsp baking soda
1/8th tsp Stevia
3 tbsp melted Raw Cacao Butter or coconut oil)
Pinch of low sodium salt
1 large pastured egg
2 tbsp coconut milk (or dairy of choice)
1 tsp pure vanilla extract
2 oz 80% cocoa bar, chopped
Top with 2 tbsp chopped nut of choice,
Optional: 1/8th tsp low sodium salt sprinkled on top of cake before baking

Chocolate Drizzle:
2 tbsp coconut cream concentrate, warmed
3 tbsp water (or coconut milk)
3 tbsp Cacao powder
1/2 tbsp pure vanilla extract
Stevia to taste

Instructions:
Preheat oven to 350 degrees F.
Oil the sides and bottom of 8 inch cake pan.
Line the bottom of the pan with parchment paper and set aside.
In a medium bowl, add dry ingredients. Use a sifter to insure that all ingredients are blended well and that there are no lumps.
Add remaining ingredients (except nuts and optional salt) to dry ingredients and mix. Taste for sweetness and adjust if necessary.
Press (or spread with angled spatula) into a 8 inch cake pan. Sprinkle with nuts. Bake for 11-14 minutes.
DO NOT OVER BAKE! Remove from oven and serve warm or allow to cool and top with Chocolate Drizzle.

Chocolate Drizzle:
In a small bowl, blend coconut cream concentrate and water until smooth.
Add cacao powder, vanilla and stevia. Whisk until creamy.
Taste for sweetness and adjust if necessary. Drizzle over the cake.

186. Choco Cookie Delight

Ingredients:
1/2 cup dark chocolate sugar free chips
1/2 cup coconut milk (thick fat from top of can)
2 eggs
1 cup almond flour
pinch of low sodium salt
1/2 teaspoon vanilla extract
1/4 teaspoon baking powder

Vanilla glaze:
1/2 cup coconut butter, liquid
Stevia to taste
1 /2 teaspoon vanilla extract

Chocolate Glaze:
1/2 cup chocolate chips
Stevia powder for decoration

Instructions:
Place a small sauce pan over low heat and melt your chocolate and coconut milk together (only keep the heat on long enough to melt them together)
While melting, place your 2 eggs in a stand mixer with the whisk, or use a hand mixer with the whisk and beat your eggs until they are fluffy, about 1 minute
Add your coconut milk and chocolate to your eggs and mix well
Stir in your almond flour, low sodium salt, vanilla extract and baking powder
Mix well ensuring everything is combined
Pipe your batter into the cookie wells ensuring you fill higher than the halfway point
Remove from the cookie maker, gently insert the sticks and place everything in the freezer for 30-45 minutes

Vanilla Glaze:
Combine your coconut butter, stevia, and vanilla extract in a small glass to make it easy to dip
You can keep this glass in hot water to keep the glaze more liquidy to make the dipping easier

Chocolate Glaze:
Melt your chocolate chips over a double boiler and keep the heat low and them liquid – then spread over cooled cookies!

187. Best Ever Banana Surprise Cake

Ingredients:
Bottom Fruit Layer:
2 tbsps coconut oil, melted
1 small banana, sliced, or ¼ cup blueberries for low carb version
2 tbsps walnut pieces * optional, can omit for nut free.
Stevia to taste
1 tsp ground cinnamon.

Top Cake Layer:
2 eggs, beaten.
Stevia to taste
¼ cup unsweetened coconut milk, or unsweetened almond milk.
1 tsp organic GF vanilla extract, or 1 tsp ground vanilla bean
½ tsp baking soda.
1 tsp apple cider vinegar.
1 small banana, mashed, or ¼ cup blueberries for lower carb version.
⅓ cup coconut flour

Instructions:
Preheat oven to 350 F, and lightly grease a 9 inch cake pan.
Place 2 tbsps coconut oil into cake pan, and put pan into preheating oven for a couple minutes to melt butter or oil. Once melted, make sure butter or oil is evenly distributed all over the bottom of the pan.
Sprinkle 2-4 drops stevia sweetener all over the melted oil.
Sprinkle 1 tsp cinnamon on top of sweetener layer.
Layer banana slices or blueberries on top of butter- sweetener layer, as seen in photo above. Add optional walnut pieces to fruit layer. Set aside.
In a large mixing bowl combine all the "top cake layer" ingredients except for the coconut flour. Mix thoroughly, then add the coconut flour and mix well, scraping sides of bowl, and braking up any coconut flour clumps.
Spoon cake batter on top of fruit layer in cake pan
Spread cake batter evenly across entire pan.
Bake for 25 minutes or until top of cake is browned and center is set.
Remove from oven and let cool completely.
Use a butter knife between cake and edge of pan and slide around to loosen cake from pan. Turn cake pan upside down onto a large plate or serving platter.
Slice and serve.
Should be stored in fridge, if serving later.

188. Coco – Walnut Brownie Bites

Ingredients:
2/3 cup raw walnut halves and pieces
1/3 cup unsweetened cocoa powder
1 tablespoon vanilla extract
1 to 2 tablespoons coconut milk
2/3 cups shredded unsweetened coconut

Instructions:

Pulse coconut in food processor for 30 seconds to a minute to form coconut crumbs. Remove from food processor and set aside.

Add unsweetened cocoa powder and walnuts to food processor, blend until walnuts become fine crumbs, but do not over process or you will get some kind of chocolate walnut butter.

Place in the food processor the cocoa walnut crumbs. Add vanilla. Process until mixture starts to combine.

Add coconut milk. You will know the consistency is right when the dough combines into a ball in the middle of the food processor.

If dough is too runny add a tablespoon or more cocoa powder to bring it back to a dough like state.

Transfer dough to a bowl and cover with plastic wrap. Refrigerate for at least 2 hours. Cold dough is much easier to work with. I left my dough in the fridge over night. You could put it in the freezer if you need to speed the process up.

Roll the dough balls in coconut crumbs, pressing the crumbs gently into the ball. Continue until all dough is gone.

189. Choco-coco Brownies

Ingredients:
6 Tablespoons of coconut oil
6 ounces of Sugar free Chocolate
4 Tablespoons of Packed Coconut Flour (20g)
¼ cup of Unsweetened Cocoa Powder (30g)
2 Eggs
½ teaspoon of Baking Soda
¼ teaspoon of low sodium salt
Extra coconut oil for pan greasing
Stevia to taste

Instructions:
Preheat the oven to 350F. Grease an 8x8 baking pan and line with parchment paper.
Ensure eggs are at room temperature. You may run them under warm water for about 10 seconds while shelled.
Gently melt the semisweet chocolate and oil in a double boiler. You may use the microwave at 50% heat at 30 second intervals with intermittent stirring.
Stir in unsweetened cocoa powder.
Sift together the superfine coconut flour, baking soda, stevia and low sodium salt.
Beat the eggs and add the dry ingredients. Beat until combined
Add the rest of the wet ingredients and beat until incorporated.
Pour the batter into the lined 8x8 pan.
Bake for 25-30 minutes at 350F until a toothpick inserted into the center of the batter comes out clean.
When done, remove from the oven and let cool in the pan for at least 15 minutes.

190. Spectacular Spinach Brownies

Ingredients:
1 ¼ cups frozen chopped spinach
6 oz sugar free chocolate
½ cup extra virgin coconut oil
½ cup coconut oil
6 eggs
Stevia to taste
½ cup cocoa powder
1 Tspn vanilla pod
¼ tsp baking soda
½ tsp low sodium salt
½ tsp cream of tartar
pinch cinnamon

Instructions:
Preheat oven to 325F. Line a 9"x13" baking pan with wax paper or use a silicone baking pan.
Melt coconut oil and chocolate together over low heat on the stove top or medium power in the microwave. Add vanilla and stir to incorporate. Let cool.
Mix cocoa powder, baking soda, cream of tartar, low sodium salt and cinnamon.
Blend spinach, egg, together in a food processor or blender, until completely smooth (2-4 minutes).
Add coconut oil to food processor and process until full incorporated.
Add melted chocolate mixture and 3 or 4 drops stevia liquid to egg mixture slowly and processing/blending constantly.
Mix in dry ingredients and process/stir to fully incorporate.
Pour batter into prepared baking pan and spread out with a spatula.
Bake for 40 minutes. Cool completely in pan. Cut into squares. Enjoy!

191. Best Banana Nut Bread

Ingredients:
3 bananas, mashed, or 1 cup
3 eggs
1/2 cup almond butter
1/4 cup coconut oil, melted
1 tsp vanilla extract
1/2 cup almond flour
1/2 cup coconut flour
2 tsp cinnamon
1 tsp baking soda
1/4 tsp low sodium salt
1/2 cup chopped walnuts
1-2 drops stevia

Instructions:
Preheat the oven to 350 degrees F. Line a loaf pan with parchment paper. In a large bowl, add the mashed bananas, eggs, almond butter, coconut oil, and vanilla. Use a hand blender to combine.
In a separate bowl, mix together the almond flour, coconut flour, cinnamon, baking soda, and low sodium salt. Blend the dry ingredients into the wet mixture, scraping down the sides with a spatula. Fold in the walnuts.
Pour the batter into the loaf pan in an even layer. Bake for 50-60 minutes, until a toothpick inserted into the center comes out clean. Place the bread on a cooling rack and allow to cool before slicing.

192. Carrot Coconut Surprise

Ingredients
1/4 cup coconut flour
2 smallish-medium-sized carrots, about 2.5 oz/70 gr each
1/4 cup almond milk
2 eggs
Low sodium salt and pepper, to taste

Instructions
1. Preheat your oven to 400 degrees and line a baking sheet with parchment paper.
2. Put the carrots and coconut in your food processor and blend for about 30-60 seconds, until the mixture looks like orange crumbs. Add everything else into the food processor and blend for about a minute or until the mixture is smooth.
3. Divide the mixture into 8 parts and form into rounds on the baking sheet. If necessary, slightly dampen your hands to flatten the rounds and prevent the dough from sticking to your hands. The rounds should be a bit thicker than 1/4 inch - not too thin, or they won't hold together.
4. Bake for about 15-17 minutes until slightly browned on the bottom and dry on the top. Let cool for a few minutes before removing from the pan.

**These biscuits are best to eat within an hour after baking, so I won't recommend to bake plenty. Bake just enough.

193. Relishing Raisin Bread

Ingredients:
- 6 room temp eggs *see tip below
- 1/3 cup melted coconut oil
- 1/3 tsp stevia
- 1/2 cup coconut milk
- 1/2 tsp vanilla extract
- 1/2 cup coconut flour
- 1 tsp cream of tartar
- 1/2 tsp baking soda
- Low sodium salt (to taste)

For the Swirl:
- 2 tbsp water
- 1/2 tbsp cinnamon
- 1 tsp stevia
- A pinch of low sodium salt (to taste)
- 1/4 cup raisins

Directions:
1. Pre-heat your oven to 325 degrees. Cover the bottom of an 8×4 loaf pan with parchment paper and grease the sides (and bottom if you do not have parchment paper) with palm shortening (or other baking fat you chose).
2. Separate the eggs – this will allow you to whip up your egg whites and ensure a good light texture. Place your egg whites in a medium, clean bowl, and set it aside. Place your egg yolks in a large mixing bowl.
3. Add the rest of the wet ingredients to your yolks. Cream until smooth.
4. Add your dry ingredients, mix until well-combined.
5. Get your cinnamon swirl ready – simply mix together the first 4 swirl ingredients in a small bowl – Keep your raisins separate.
6. With a hand mixer or KitchenAid mixer – using clean beaters – on a medium speed whip up your egg whites until soft peaks begin to form when you remove the beaters. Fold the egg whites into the batter until just combined.
7. Add about 1/3 of the batter to your loaf pan – drizzle 1/2 of your swirl, and then quickly with a knife lightly zig-zag the swirl on top of the batter. Sprinkle with half of your raisins
8. Add another third of the batter and drizzle the rest of the swirl.
9. Top with rest of batter.
10. Place in oven to cook for 47-50 minutes – until the top is bouncy or until when a toothpick is inserted in the top it comes out clean.
11. Remove and let cool for 5-10 minutes. Flip out to complete cooling. Can be tightly wrapped and stored on counter for 5-7 days, or placed in fridge for 10-14 days.

194. Luscious Lemon Delight

Ingredients:
- 6 eggs
- 1/4 cup coconut oil, melted
- zest from 2 lemons
- 1/3 cup lemon juice
- 1 cup milk (almond or coconut)
- 2/3 cup coconut flour (do not substitute another flour)
- 1 heaping teaspoon baking soda
- Pinch of low sodium salt (to taste)

Lemon Glaze:
- 2 Tbsp coconut oil
- 1 tbsp water
- 1 tsp stevia
- 2 Tbsp almond milk
- zest and juice from 1 lemon
- 1/2 tsp pure vanilla extract

Directions:
1. Preheat oven to 350 F.
2. Combine all bread ingredients in a mixing bowl and mix well. Pour into a greased pan and bake for 32-45 minutes or until golden on top and the middle is cooked through. Remove from oven and let cool.
3. While the lemon loaf is baking, mix all glaze ingredients together in a small pot over low heat until it starts to simmer. Remove from heat and let sit to cool until the lemon loaf is finished cooking and cooling. Pour the glaze all over the top of the loaf. Refrigerate the loaf at least 30 minutes – 1 hour until both the glaze and the loaf firms up a bit.
4. Enjoy! You can store leftovers in the refrigerator for up to 3 days.

195. Sexy Sweet Potato

Ingredients
300 grams cooked sweet potato flesh*
1/2 cup coconut flour
3 eggs
3 tablespoons of coconut milk
1 teaspoon baking soda
Juice of half a lemon
A pinch of low sodium salt

*I roast a purple skin / white flesh sweet potato and keep the flesh for this recipe, I personally think the skins are delicious ad eat them as they are. You can use whatever sweet potato you like.

Instructions
1. Preheat your oven to 180 Degrees Celsius or 350 Degrees Fahrenheit.
2. Grease and line a mini loaf tin (mine is 6" x 2.5") with baking paper hanging over the sides for easy removal.
3. Put the ingredients into your food processor or blender and pulse until well combined. Spoon the mixture into the prepared tin, smooth over the top with a spoon. Bake for 40 minutes. Cover the loaf with foil and bake for a further 20 minutes. Remove from the oven and allow the bread to cool before slicing. Enjoy.

196. Cheeky Coconut Loaf

Ingredients
1/2 cup coconut flour, sifted
3 eggs
zest of one lemon
1/2 cup desiccated coconut
1 cup coconut yoghurt
1 teaspoon ground cardamom
¼ cup almond milk
2 tsp stevia
A pinch of low sodium salt
1/2 teaspoon concentrated natural vanilla extract
1 teaspoon baking soda
Instructions
1. Preheat your oven to 175 degrees Celsius or 350 degrees Fahrenheit
2. Grease a mini loaf tin (mine is 16cm x 6cm)
3. Combine the flour, zest, coconut, baking soda and cardamom. Add the eggs, mix together. Add the yoghurt, milk and stevia, combine. Add the salt and vanilla, combine. Spoon the mixture into your prepared pan. Bake for 35 minutes. Cover with foil and bake for another 10 minutes. Remove from the oven and allow it to cool slightly before flipping onto a cooling tray. Leave to cool for a few minutes before cutting into thick slices.
4. This is great toasted and served with butter. Enjoy.

197. Heavenly Herb Flatbread

Ingredients:
1/2 cup Coconut Flour
3 eggs
1 cup coconut milk or almond milk
1/2 tsp low sodium salt
1/2 tsp dried oregano
1/2 tsp dried basil
1/2 tsp garlic powder
drizzle of coconut oil

Instructions
1. Preheat oven to 375 degrees.
2. Mix together the coconut flour, salt, herbs, & garlic powder in a bowl.
3. Whisk the eggs and coconut milk in a separate bowl.
4. Pour the wet ingredients into the coconut flour mixture.
5. Stir until no lumps are left. Let the batter sit for at least 5 minutes (so the coconut flour absorbs all the liquid). It should resemble a thick paste.
6. Prepare your pan. Drizzle some coconut oil on the bottom of pan (10 x 15 " rimmed pan) and then place the parchment paper (oil first helps the corners stick). I also drizzled some coconut oil on top of the paper and spread it out with a pastry brush.
7. Pour out all the mixture into the pan. Tap the pan until the upper part is flat. (this will help your bread to cook evenly)
8. Cook for 30- 40 minutes or until the toothpick comes out clean.
9. Allow the bread to cool before transferring it to your container or serving plate.

198. Cozy Coconut Flour Muffins

Ingredients
1/2 cup coconut flour
6 eggs, at room temperature (that's important)
¼ cup almond milk
2 tsp stevia
6 Tbs. coconut oil
2 Tbsp coconut milk at room temperature
2 tsp. vanilla extract
1/4 tsp. baking soda
1 tsp. apple cider vinegar

Instructions
1. Preheat the oven to 350 degrees and prepare a muffin tin with 8 liners (I like unbleached parchment paper baking cups).
2. Combine the coconut flour and eggs until smooth. Add the remaining ingredients and stir well.
3. Divide evenly between the muffin tins. Bake until golden and a toothpick comes out clean, about 20 minutes.
4. Cool completely.

**Makes 8 cupcakes. Feel free to double the recipe if you want more cupcakes! These last in an airtight container for a few days at room temperature. They also freeze really well!

199. Naked Chocolate Cake

Ingredients
1/2 cup (2 3/4 oz) Naked Chocolate or a good quality cocoa
1/2 cup (2 3/4 oz) coconut flour
2 1/2 teaspoons gluten free baking powder
1/2 teaspoon ground cinnamon
Pinch of low sodium salt
6 free-range eggs
1/2 cup (4 1/2 fl oz) coconut oil
3/4 cup coconut milk
1 teaspoon stevia
1 teaspoon vanilla paste

Instructions:
Preheat oven to 160°C (320°F)
1. Combine the cocoa, coconut flour, baking powder, cinnamon and salt into a mixing bowl.
2. Add the eggs, stevia, vanilla, coconut milk and coconut oil.
3. Mix well until smooth and combined – a whisk works well for this.
4. Pour into a 20 cm (9 inch) baking tin lined with baking paper.
5. Bake the cake for 55 – 60 minutes or until cooked through. Best to test after 45 to make sure as oven temps may vary.
6. Remove from the oven and cool.
7. Spread with ganache or healthy chocolate mousse and enjoy.

200. Blueberry Sponge Roll Surprise

Ingredients
6 eggs, separated
1/3 cup almond milk
1/2 cup coconut flour
1/2 teaspoon baking soda
1/4 teaspoon vanilla powder
1 tsp stevia

For filling:
1 can coconut cream (chilled in fridge overnight)
¼ cup blueberry
A few drops of stevia

Instructions:
1. Heat oven to 170 degrees Celsius (338F)
2. Line a 24 x 30cm (base measurement) Swiss roll pan with baking paper.
3. Beat egg whites with electric beaters until they form soft peaks.
4. In a separate bowl, beat egg yolks and honey until pale yellow. (1-2 mins)
5. Add coconut flour, vanilla powder and baking soda to yolks, add milk and stevia and beat until well combined.
6. Using a metal spoon, mix 1/3 of the egg white mixture into the egg & flour mixture.
7. Gently fold in the remaining egg whites.
8. Spread into lined pan and bake for 12-15 mins until golden brown.
9. When cake comes out of the oven, lift it from the pan using the baking paper.
10. Leaving the cake on the paper, start from the short end and roll the cake into a log.
11. Place in fridge to cool with seam side down.
12. While cake is cooling, use electric beaters to beat the coconut cream that has separated to the top of the can and put a few drops of stevia on it. (About 1 cup) After doing the cream, slice blueberries into small pieces.
13. After cake has cooled, unroll and spread the coconut cream and put sliced blueberries at the   top of the cake.
14. Using the paper as a guide, re-roll again from the short side.
15. Sprinkle top with coconut flour if you like.
16. Serve straight away, or store in the fridge.

Paleo Diet Recipes 365 Days of Paleo and Coconut Recipes by Mercedes Del Rey

201. Lemon Mousse Mouthwatering Cupcakes

Ingredients
1/2 cup coconut flour
6 eggs, at room temperature (that's important)
6 Tbs. milk
2 tsp stevia
6 Tbs. coconut oil
2 Tbs. coconut milk at room temperature
1 tsp. vanilla extract
1/2 tsp. ground cardamom
1/4 tsp. baking soda
1/2 tsp. apple cider vinegar

Instructions
1. Preheat the oven to 350 degrees and prepare a muffin tin with 8 liners (I like unbleached parchment paper baking cups).
2. Combine the coconut flour and eggs until smooth. Add the remaining ingredients and stir well.
3. Divide evenly between the muffin tins. Bake until golden and a toothpick comes out clean, about 20 minutes.
4. Cool completely and frost with the lemon mousse.
5. Makes 8 cupcakes. Feel free to double the recipe if you want more cupcakes!

Lemon Mousse Frosting
Ingredients
3/4 cup stevia-sweetened lemon curd (recipe below)
1 cup coconut milk
1 Tbs. light coconut milk
1 tsp stevia
Pinch of salt to taste

Instructions
1. First, make the stevia-sweetened lemon curd, by simply whisking the whole eggs, yolks and 1tsp stevia in a saucepan until smooth, then place pan over a low heat. Add the coconut oil, juice and zest and whisk continuously until thickened. Strain through a sieve. Lemon curd keeps, covered, in the fridge for 2 weeks. Chill until thickened and cold before using it.
2. In a small saucepan, whisk together the coconut milk and gelatin. Let it sit for 10 minutes. Then turn the heat on medium and whisk until the gelatin dissolves. Pour into a bowl and refrigerate until set, about 4 hours.
3. In a food processor, blend together the set coconut milk and the lemon curd until smooth. Add stevia to taste and a small pinch of salt.

202. Chocolate Raspberry Cake Delight

Ingredients
For the cake
1/2 cup (120g) of Coconut Oil
1/4 cup (30g) of Coconut Flour
1/3 cup (45g) of Arrowroot Starch
1/4 cup (35g) of Unsweetened Cocoa Powder
1 teaspoon of Baking Soda
1/4 cup almond milk
1/4 cup of Strong Hot Coffee
1 tbsp Stevia
4 large Eggs
1 teaspoon of Vanilla Extract
For the raspberry sauce
10 ounces of Raspberries
1 teaspoon of Lemon Juice
1/4 cup almond milk
1 tsp Stevia
1/2 teaspoon of Gelatin
For the chocolate ganache
3 ounces of Chocolate Chips
1/3 cup of Full Fat Coconut Milk

Instructions
1. FOR THE CAKE: Whip together the coconut oil and stevia in a large mixer until combined, about 3 minutes on high speed.
2. Sift together the coconut flour, arrowroot flour, cocoa powder, and baking soda in a separate bowl. Whisk together the eggs, milk, stevia, coffee, and extract in a large glass.
3. Add about a third of the dry ingredients and a third of the liquid ingredients to the mixing bowl and mix until combined. Repeat adding the ingredients in batches until all mixed and uniform.
4. Evenly portion the cake batter into muffin tin cups. Bake at 350F for 25-28 minutes, until an inserted toothpick comes out clean.
5. Remove from the oven and let the cakes cool for about 10 minutes. Gently remove the cakes from the tin cups using a rubber spatula and set on a cooling rack upside down.
FOR THE RASPBERRY SAUCE: Reserve a few raspberries for garnish.
Gently heat the raspberries, lemon juice, and milk and stevia for about 5 minutes. Remove from heat when the mixture looks uniform. Sprinkle the gelatin on the jam and mix until dissolved.
FOR THE CHOCOLATE GANACHE
Heat the coconut milk to a very low boil. Add to the half of the chocolate chips and mix until fully combined. Then add the rest and mix until uniform. Let cool to a thick yet pourable consistency before use.
   ASSEMBLY: Scoop out a portion of cupcake from the center, careful not to puncture it completely. Fill the hole with about a tablespoon of the raspberry sauce. Pour about 2 tablespoons worth directly on top of the raspberry center.

  * *Use a frosting spatula or the back of a spoon to spread the chocolate in a circular motion toward the cupcake edges. Let the chocolate goodness fall to the sides. Top with a raspberry and enjoy!

Paleo Diet Recipes 365 Days of Paleo and Coconut Recipes by Mercedes Del Rey

203. Strawberry Dashing Doughnuts

Ingredients:
4 large eggs, room temperature
3 tablespoons coconut oil, melted
¾ cup coconut milk, warm
1 tsp Stevia
1 teaspoon apple cider vinegar
1 teaspoon pure vanilla extract
½ cup coconut flour
¼ cup strawberries, grind
½ teaspoon baking soda
¼ teaspoon low sodium salt

Topping
1 ounce raw cacao butter, melted
2 tablespoons coconut butter
1 teaspoon stevia
¼ cup strawberries, grind

Instructions:
1. Preheat a doughnut maker. If using a doughnut pan, preheat the oven to 350F and grease the pan liberally with butter.
2. Using a stand mixer or electric hand mixer, beat the eggs with the coconut oil on medium-high speed until creamy.
3. Add the milk, stevia, vinegar, and vanilla and beat again until combined.
4. Using a fine mesh sieve or sifter, sift the remaining dry ingredients into the bowl. Beat on high until smooth.
5. Scoop the batter into a large Ziploc bag, seal the top, and snip one of the bottom corners.
6. Pipe the batter into the doughnut mold, filling it completely.
7. Cook until the doughnut machine indicator light goes off. If you are using an oven, bake for 17 minutes. Remove the doughnuts and cool on a wire rack. Trim if necessary.

Make the glaze
1. Mix the cacao butter, coconut butter, and stevia in a shallow bowl. Place in the freezer for 5 minutes to thicken.
2. Once the donuts are completely cooled, sprinkle ground strawberries on top.
3. Place in the refrigerator for 20 minutes to allow the glaze to set.

204. Perfect Plantain Cake Surprise

Ingredients
4 eggs, separated
2 tsp cream of tartar
1/2 cup extra virgin coconut oil
1/4 cup almond milk
2 tsp Stevia
1 cup ripe plantain, mashed (equals one plantain)
4 tsp vanilla extract
1/2 cup coconut flour, sifted
1/2 tsp baking soda
1/4 tsp low sodium salt

Instructions
1. Preheat oven to 350 degrees F. In a bowl combine egg whites and cream of tartar.
2. Whip the egg whites until stiff peaks form.
3. In a separate bowl cream together coconut oil, stevia and milk. Do that for a few minutes.
4. Add the egg yolks. Mix until smooth. Add mashed plantain and vanilla until mixed.
5. Add the sifted coconut flour, baking soda and salt to the egg yolk mixture. Mix until smooth. Slowly add the egg yolk mixture to the whipped egg whites.
6. Line an 8 x 1.5 inch cake tin with parchment paper and grease the sides.
7. Bake for 35 minutes until the top is firm to the touch and a toothpick can be inserted and comes out dry.

205. Lemon Blueberry Cake Delight

Ingredients
½ cup coconut flour, sifted
3 eggs, beaten
⅓ cup unsweetened coconut milk or almond milk
2 tbsp lemon juice, (use lemon squeezer to get all the juice)
1 tbsp lemon zest
2 ½ tbsp. coconut oil, melted
½ tbsp liquid stevia
1 tsp lemon extract (organic GF kind).
½ tsp baking soda + 1 tsp apple cider vinegar, mixed in separate pinch bowl (should be very fizzy)
½ cup blueberries *optional.
Lemon Ice Glaze:
2 tbsp coconut oil, melted
1½ tbsp coconut butter, melted
1 ½ tbsp unsweetened coconut milk
1½ tbsp lemon juice
½ tsp lemon extract (organic GF kind)
2 tsp lemon zest
1/3 tsp liquid stevia (as sweetener)
Instructions
1. Preheat oven to 350 F, and grease or oil a 9" round cake pan.
2. In a large mixing bowl combine: all the first 8 cake ingredients. Stir together thoroughly; break up any coconut flour lumps. Add in baking soda and vinegar mixture and stir.
3. Gently add and mix in the blueberries.
4. Spoon cake batter into prepared pan and spread around evenly.
5. Bake in 350 F oven for 30 minutes or until center is firm.
6. Remove cake from oven and let cool for 10 minutes while you make the lemon ice glaze.
7. Heat a small sauce pan over low heat and melt: coconut oil, and coconut butter. Stir the mixture as it melts and break up any coconut butter lumps.
8. Once melted, remove from heat and add all the rest of the lemon ice glaze ingredients. Stir the glaze thoroughly until well mixed and set aside to cool.
9. Use a metal or wooden skewer, or large toothpick to poke holes all over the cake. Be sure to poke all the way down to the bottom of cake.
10. Spoon or pour lemon ice glaze all over the top of cake, making sure to cover well. Use the back of a spoon to spread around evenly.
11. Let cake cool and glaze set awhile. It should only take 5 minutes or so for glaze to solidify a bit.
12. Slice and serve. Unused portions should be stored in the fridge.

206. Delicious Coconut Flour Cake with Strawberry Surprise

Ingredients
1 dozen eggs
2 cups coconut milk (I used homemade)
¼ cup milk
2 teaspoons Stevia
2 teaspoons vanilla extract
2 cups coconut flour
1/2 teaspoon baking soda
1/4 teaspoon low sodium salt
coconut oil for greasing the pan

Instruction
1. Preheat oven to 350F.
2. Whisk together the eggs, coconut milk, milk, stevia and vanilla extract. Mix until smooth.
3. Add coconut flour, baking soda and salt to the egg mixture and whisk until a smooth batter forms.
4. Grease 2 – 9 inch round cake pans with coconut oil.
5. Divide up the batter evenly between the 2 cake tins. Use a rubber spatula to smooth it out.
6. Bake for 40 minutes, or until a toothpick inserted into the center of the cake comes out clean.
7. Allow the cake to cool.
8. Fill the center with cooked strawberries (recipe below). You can also use the strawberry filling to decorate the cake.

Strawberry Filling
Ingredients
2 cups organic strawberries, stems removed and sliced
1. Place the strawberries in a saucepan over medium heat.
2. After a few minutes, the strawberries will release their juices.
3. Allow them to cook uncovered, occasionally stirring and smashing them.
4. Keep cooking them until the strawberries are soft, smashed and the sauce has reduced. About 30 minutes.

207. Titillating Berry Trifle

Ingredients:
1/2 cup plus 2 tsp coconut flour, sifted
1/4 tsp low sodium salt
1/4 tsp baking soda
5 whole eggs (2 of them separated)
1/2 cup coconut oil, softened
1/2 cup almond milk
2 tsp stevia
1 tablespoon vanilla extract
2 teaspoons lemon juice
1 1/2-2 cups washed & diced strawberries (cut large if using a traditional Trifle bowl)
1 1/2-2 cups washed blueberries
1 1/2-2 cups washed raspberries
3-4 cans full-fat coconut milk, cream only

Instruction:
1. Preheat oven to 350 degrees.
2. Sift the dry ingredients together and set aside.
3. Separate 2 of the eggs, setting the whites aside and putting the 2 yolks in a medium sized bowl. Crack open the rest of the eggs, adding them to the bowl with egg yolks.
4. Using a mixer or hand whisk, beat the coconut oil (liquid or solid, doesn't matter), milk, vanilla and lemon juice until they are well combined.
5. On low/medium-speed, mix the dry ingredients into the wet ingredients. Continue to mix till the batter is smooth and has no lumps.
6. Add the eggs (not including the 2 egg whites) in three phases to the batter. Allow each addition to be incorporated completely before adding the next.
7. In a small bowl, beat the egg whites till thick soft peaks form. Fold into the batter.
8. Pour the batter into a greased 8 inch square brownie pan or 7X10 small casserole dish lined with parchment paper, allow a few inches of flaps to hang over the two long sides of the pan. This will help later with removing the cake ensure that the sides of the cake won't stick to the pan. Alternatively, you could make cup cakes with the batter and cube those up for the trifle. Baking times will vary depending on the depth of the cake pan. I find that a 1 or 2 inch high cake produces the best texture instead of a thicker cake. However, I have made this in a standard size bread pan as well, and it turns out very nice.
9. Bake for 30-45 min. or until a toothpick in the center comes out clean.
10. Allow the cake to cool for 5-10 minutes, run a sharp knife along the edges and carefully remove from the pan. Cool completely.

For the coconut whipped cream:
1. Chill 2-3 three cans of full-fat coconut milk (a few hours or overnight).
2. Open the cans and scoop the thick cream in to a medium bowl. Try to keep as much coconut liquid out of the cream as possible. Discard the liquid or freeze it into ice cube trays to use in smoothies.
3. With a hand/stand mixer, beat the cream on high for a minute or so. Add ½ tsp. stevia as sweetener if desired. Continue beating until well combined.

Assembling the Trifle:
 Assembly is super easy. Just add some cake to the bottom of your dish, then whipped cream, strawberries/raspberries, whipped cream, more cake, blueberries, more whipped cream, then more fruit if desired or cake crumbles. Really just layer it however you like!

This recipe should make enough for 4 individual 12 oz trifles or you can make two cakes, add extra fruit and more coconut cream (2-3 more cans) for one, 2-quart trifle or glass bowl.

208. Lemon-Coconut Petit Fours

Ingredients
For the Cake
1/2 cup coconut flour
1/2 cup coconut milk
3 eggs, separated
3/4 cup soaked dates in 3 tbsp hot water
1/2 tsp vanilla
1/2 tsp baking soda
1/4 tsp low sodium salt
1 tsp lemon rind

Frosting
2/3 cup coconut cream (from the top of a can of coconut milk)
2 tbsp almond milk
1 tbsp Stevia
3 tsp lemon juice
¼ cup coconut oil, room temperature

Instructions
1. Put dates in a heat safe bowl or container and pour 3 tbsp boiling water over them and let soak for about 15 minutes. You can chop the dates before soaking to speed up the process, but it's not necessary.
2. Separate the eggs with yolks in one bowl and whites in one large stainless steel, glass or ceramic bowl. When you go to whip the egg whites, it helps if they are at room temperature.
3. Once dates have soaked put them in a food processor along with remaining water and mix until you have a paste-like consistency. Add coconut flour, milk, egg yolks, vanilla, baking soda, salt and lemon rind and mix.
4. Whip the egg whites until foamy and stiff peaks form. This is much easier if you have a stand mixer with the whisk attachment or a hand mixer. It is possible to do it by hand, but takes time.
5. Gently fold egg whites into the batter. Grease a standard sized loaf pan. Put batter in pan and even out the top with a spatula or spoon.
6. Bake in a 350° oven for 20-30 minutes or when a toothpick inserted comes out clean.
For the frosting
7. Coconut cream can be purchased in cans or you can skim the cream of the top of cans of coconut milk, however you may have to use multiple cans of coconut milk. Put coconut cream in a bowl and whisk for a few minutes to make it lighter and creamier.
8. Add coconut oil, milk, stevia and lemon juice and whisk until fully incorporated.
9. Allow the cake to cool completely before frosting. Once the cake has cooled, cut small squares or circles out of the cake and skim some cake off of the top with a knife to make it even. There will be leftover scraps, but they make a great snack!
10. Cut the squares in half and frost the middle. You can use the prepared frosting, but it will be very thin.
11. Drizzle the prepared frosting over the small cake squares and use a spatula or knife to frost the sides evenly. Once you've frosted each petit fours, refrigerate to allow the frosting to harden. Top with a bit of lemon rind.

209. Gingerbread Cream Delight

Ingredients
For the Gingerbread Cake
½ cup (80g) of packed Coconut Flour
½ cup (64g) of Arrowroot Flour
1 teaspoon of Baking Powder
½ teaspoon of Baking Soda
½ teaspoon of low sodium Salt
1½ teaspoon of Ginger Powder
1½ teaspoon of Cinnamon
¼ teaspoon of Nutmeg
Pinch of Cloves
½ cup of almond milk
1 teaspoon of Vanilla Extract
4 Eggs, room temperature
½ cup (100g) of Coconut Oil (softened solid)
2 tsp Stevia
For the Cream Cheese Frosting
8 oz Cream Cheese, room temperature
4 oz of Coconut oil at room temperature
2 tbsp Stevia
¼ cup of Arrowroot Flour

Instructions
For the Gingerbread Cake
1. Preheat oven to 350F and grease an 8"x4" loaf pan.
2. Sift together the coconut flour, arrowroot flour, baking powder, baking soda, salt, and spices in a bowl to form the dry mixture.
3. Combine the milk and vanilla extract in another bowl to form the liquid mixture.
4. Separate the eggs whites from the egg yolks.
5. Beat the egg whites at high speed in a mixer bowl with a whisk attachment until a meringue forms. Remove the whites from the mixer bowl and set aside.
6. Add the coconut oil and coconut sugar to the mixing bowl and beat on medium high for about a minute until uniform.
7. Add the egg yolks one at a time to the mixing bowl and beat on medium until combined. Scrape the sides if necessary.
8. Add half of the dry mixture to the mixing bowl and beat until combined.
9. Add half of the liquid mixture to the mixing bowl and beat.
10. Repeat the previous two steps until all mixed.
11. Portion a heaping of the egg whites and add to the mixing bowl and mix.
12. Fold in the rest of the egg whites until uniform.
13. Pour batter into the loaf pan and bake, centered rack, at 350F for 35-40 minutes.

For the Frosting
1. Whip the coconut oil and cream cheese until smooth.
2. Add the arrowroot flour and stevia.
3. Whip on low until the flour is absorbed into the butter, then whip on high for a few minutes until light and fluffy.

210. Mouthwatering Coconut Custard Cake

Ingredients:
4 eggs
2 ½ cups almond milk
1/2 cup coconut flour
1 tsp pure vanilla extract
2 tsp baking powder
2 tsp stevia
1/4 cup coconut, melted
1 1/2 cups unsweetened, coconut flakes
1/2 cup chocolate chips or broken chocolate bar

Instruction
1. Pre-heat oven to 350F.
2. In a large bowl of a stand mixer (or whisk by hand) eggs, milk, coconut flour, stevia, vanilla, coconut oil, and baking powder until smooth.
3. Stir in coconut flakes and chocolate.
4. Pour into an 8" cake pan and bake for 45 - 50 minutes or until a toothpick inserted into middle comes out clean.
5. Allow to cool before slicing in pan, and serving.
6. Sprinkle with cinnamon just before serving.

211. Cranberry Orange Upside Down Revolution

Fruit:
unbleached parchment paper
2 cups fresh cranberries
1 tablespoon coconut oil (at room temperature)
1 teaspoon stevia
1 tablespoon arrowroot powder

Dry Ingredients:
6 tablespoons coconut flour
6 tablespoons arrowroot powder
2 teaspoons baking powder
1/4 teaspoon low sodium salt

Wet Ingredients:
4 large pastured eggs
4 tablespoons melted coconut oil
4 tablespoons almond milk
2 tablespoons freshly squeezed orange juice
A zest of 1 organic orange
1 teaspoon vanilla

Instruction
1. Preheat oven to 350 degrees F. Place a 9-inch cake pan onto a sheet of parchment paper and draw a line around the bottom with a pencil. Cut out the circle and place it onto the bottom of the cake pan. Grease the sides of the pan with coconut oil.
2. In a small bowl mix together the coconut oil, milk, and arrowroot powder. Spread it onto the parchment paper in the cake pan (I use an offset spatula to do this). Arrange the cranberries on top of the mixture.
3. Whisk together the dry ingredients. In a separate bowl, whisk together the wet ingredients. Pour the wet into the dry and quickly whisk together until combined. Pour batter over fruit and spread evenly with the back of a spoon or spatula.
4. Bake for 30 to 35 minutes. Let pan cool on a wire rack for 15 to 20 minutes then carefully flip out onto a plate; peel off parchment paper. Let cool and then serve. Enjoy!

212. Baked Vanilla Cardamom Delights

Ingredients:
1/2 cup coconut flour
1/8 teaspoon baking soda
3/4 teaspoon baking powder
1/4 cup Stevia liquid drops
1/4-1/2 teaspoon cardamom (we did 1/2 because we love cardamom)
2 egg, room temperature
2 tablespoons coconut oil, liquid (or oil of choice)
1/2 cup warm water

Instructions:
1. In a bowl place all dry ingredients into bowl and whisk together. Set aside.
2. Next grab your stevia, coconut oil and egg and whisk together in mixing bowl. Once that is all mixed together add in your dry ingredients. Begin to stir the donut batter.
3. End with adding in your warm water to the batter and stir till smooth and combined.
4. Pre-heat your mini donut maker. Once your green light turns off it is ready. Begin to scoop your donut batter into each mini donut ring. We used a cookie scooper to help with the scooping.
5. Once all rings are filled close the donut maker and let bake for 2-3 minutes. Check and see if they feel done. If so remove carefully with a knife. Repeat process till all our donut batter has been baked.
6. Remove donuts from pan with a knife. Serve and enjoy.

213. Pumpkin Cream Cookies

Ingredients
For the donuts
- 6 dried medjool dates, pitted
- ½ cup pumpkin puree
- ¼ cup coconut oil, melted
- 4 eggs
- 3 tablespoons coconut flour
- ½ tablespoon cinnamon
- ¼ teaspoon nutmeg
- ⅛ teaspoon ground cloves
- ⅛ teaspoon ground ginger
- ½ teaspoon baking powder
- A pinch of low sodium salt

For the cream
- 1 (14 ounce) can of coconut cream OR coconut milk refrigerated overnight*
- 1 tablespoon stevia
- ¼ teaspoon cinnamon

For the chocolate
- 1 cup Enjoy Life Chocolate Chips, melted
- 3 tablespoons coconut milk

Instructions
1. Place dried dates in a food processor and pulse to break down.
2. Add pumpkin puree, melted coconut oil, and eggs to the food processor and puree until smooth.
3. Add coconut flour, cinnamon, nutmeg, ground cloves, ginger, baking powder, and a pinch of salt and puree once more.
*To make the donuts easy to pour and keep them a round shape, place donut puree into a plastic bag or pastry bag, cut the end off of the plastic bag so you can squeeze to mixture in a circle in the donut maker. If you are using a donut pan for the oven, preheat oven to 350 degrees.
4. Heat up a mini donut maker, grease the donut maker or pan, and use the bag to squeeze about 2 tablespoons of the mixture into each donut round.
5. In a mini donut maker, cook for 5-7 minutes. Times will vary with the different donut maker. If you are using a donut pan, cook for 20-25 minutes.
6. Remove donuts once cooked through and let rest and cool on a wire rack.
7. Once cooled, place in refrigerator for about 10 minutes. (The donuts will be easier to work with once they are a bit harder).
8. While the donuts cool, in a bowl, remove the coconut cream that sits on top of the coconut water (keep the coconut water for later) and whip together the coconut cream with a fork or whisk. Then add maple syrup and cinnamon and mix well. Place cream in a piping bag or plastic bag and then cut off the end.
9. In a bowl, melt chocolate chips and coconut milk that was left behind from the coconut cream via a double boiler or in a microwave.
10. Cut the donuts in half, carefully. On the bottom donut, pipe on the cream around the donut then place the top donut half on top of the cream. Then finish the donuts off by dipping them halfway into the melted chocolate.
11. Place donuts on a parchment lined baking sheet and into the freezer to harden the chocolate.
12. Once chocolate has hardened, eat up! Makes 8 mini donuts.

214. Sexy Savory Muffins

Ingredients
½ cup coconut flour
1 tsp baking soda
½-1 tsp low sodium salt
¼ cup coconut oil
½ cup + 2 tbsp coconut milk
4 pastured eggs
1 tsp apple cider vinegar
1 tsp garlic powder
½ tsp each of rosemary, thyme, sage

Instructions
1. Pre-heat the oven to 350°. Melt the coconut oil and combine with remaining muffin ingredients in a food processor or bowl, mix well.
2. Place batter in a muffin tin lined with muffin liners. The muffins will raise a small amount, so you can fill the muffin liner about ¾ full–almost to the top. Bake for about 20-30 minutes or until a toothpick inserted comes out clean and the tops are slightly browned.
3. Let it cool and slice in small squares.

215. Delicious Lady Fingers

Ingredients
4 Pastured Eggs, separated
1/4 cup almond milk
1/4 tsp Baking Soda
1/2 tsp Pure Vanilla Extract
1/3 cup Coconut Flour, sifted
1 tsp freshly ground Coffee

Instructions
1. Preheat oven to back at 400 degrees.
2. Beat egg whites until stiff in a standing kitchen mixer, or with a hand mixer.
3. In a medium sized mixing bowl, combine egg yolks, baking soda, vanilla extract, and milk. Whisk until combined.
4. Sift in the coconut flour, and continue to whisk until smooth.
5. Fold in the egg whites, followed by the coffee grounds.
6. On a parchment lined baking sheet pipe out 3 inch long cookies with a round piping tube.
7. Bake at 400 degrees for 13 minutes, or until cookies are golden brown.
8. Allow to cool and enjoy.

216. Cheeky Coconut Chocolate Cookies

Ingredients
1/2 cup Virgin Coconut Oil, melted
1/4 tsp stevia
1/2 tablespoon vanilla extract
4 eggs
1/8 teaspoon low sodium salt
1 cup coconut flour
1/2 cup shredded coconut
3/4 cup chocolate chips

Instruction
1. Preheat oven to 375 degrees F.
2. Mix together coconut oil, sugar, vanilla, eggs, and salt together. Blend thoroughly. Add flour, coconut and chocolate chips; mix thoroughly.
3. Form into small cookies on a parchment lined pan and bake in preheated oven for about 15 minutes, or until lightly browned.

217. Scrumptious Peanut Butter Parcels

Ingredients:
½ cup sifted coconut flour
1 cup natural peanut butter
½ cup peanuts, coarsely chopped (optional)
1 tsp Stevia Drops
4 eggs
½ teaspoon vanilla
½ teaspoon low sodium salt

Directions:
1. Mix together peanut butter, sugar, eggs, vanilla and salt. Stir in peanuts and coconut flour. Batter will be runny.
2. Drop by the spoonful 2 inches apart on greased cookie sheet. Bake at 375 Degrees F for about 14 minutes.
3. Cool slightly and remove from cookie sheet.

**Makes about 3 dozen cookies.

218. Chocolaty Pumpkin Muffins

Ingredients
⅓ cup pumpkin puree
⅓ cup almond milk
¼ cup coconut oil, melted
3 eggs, whisked
1 teaspoon vanilla extract
¼ cup coconut flour
½ teaspoon cinnamon
¼ teaspoon nutmeg
⅛ teaspoon ground cloves
⅛ teaspoon powdered ginger
½ teaspoon baking soda
½ teaspoon baking powder
pinch of low sodium salt
½ cup Enjoy Life Mini Chocolate Chips
1 tsp stevia

Instructions
1. Preheat oven to 350 degrees.
2. Mix together wet ingredients in a bowl: pumpkin puree, milk, coconut oil, eggs, and vanilla extract.
3. In another bowl, whisk together coconut flour, cinnamon, nutmeg, ground cloves, powdered ginger, baking soda, baking powder, and salt.
4. Pour dry ingredients into wet ingredients and mix well.
5. Fold in chocolate chips.
6. Use an ice cream scoop to scoop batter into 5 silicone baking cups.
7. Bake for 35-40 minutes

219. Succulent Shortbread Cookies

Ingredients:
3/4 cup + 1/2 cup extra coconut flour
1/4 cup arrowroot starch
1/2 cup coconut oil or butter, melted
1/8 tsp low sodium salt
5 tablespoons milk
1 tsp stevia
1/4 cup dark chocolate chips

Instruction
1. Preheat oven to 350 degrees.
2. Combine all ingredients except chocolate and 1/2 c extra coconut flour in a mixing bowl. Mush up with a fork and add additional coconut flour until the mixture is crumbly.
3. Dust a clean, smooth surface with coconut flour. Press the crumbly mixture out with your fingers to make it smooth and somewhat flat. Dust with coconut flour.
4. Roll the dough to about 1/8-1/4 inch thickness using a rolling pin. Cut shapes out of the dough. Roll the scraps up into a ball and flatten to cut more shapes out.
5. Bake on a lightly greased cookie sheet for 15 minutes. Allow the cookies to cool.
6. Microwave the chocolate chips for 10 second intervals, stirring between intervals, until they are melted. Drizzle cookies with the chocolate. If the chocolate is not very runny, add a tiny amount of coconut oil and stir.
7. Allow the cookies to cool in the fridge or freezer for a few minutes until the chocolate is set.

220. Tasty Coconut Pancakes

Ingredients:
1/4 cup coconut flour
1/8 tsp baking soda
Pinch of low sodium salt
1/3 - 1/4 cup coconut milk
2 tbsp organic, cold-pressed coconut oil
3 eggs
1 tsp stevia
1/2 tsp vanilla extract
Coconut oil for cooking

Instruction
1. Thoroughly mix the eggs, coconut oil, and stevia together.
2. Add the coconut milk and vanilla extract.
3. Throw in the coconut flour, baking soda, and salt. Mix, but remember, not too much!
4. Place a little coconut oil in your skillet and then using a measuring cup, add a little batter to the pan. I recommend figuring out how many pancakes you'd like to make beforehand so that you can use an appropriately sized cup or ladle. This recipe should yield around 8 or so pancakes.
5. Remember that you aren't likely to see many bubbles forming on the top, so carefully check the underside of your pancake before flipping.
6. For best results, serve your pancakes with Blueberry sauce

Blueberry Sauce

Ingredients
2 cups fresh or frozen blueberries (no need to thaw before use if frozen)
1/4 cup water
2 tsp. arrowroot powder
1 Tbs. water

Instruction
1. Place the berries and 1/4 cup water (or juice) in a small saucepan over medium heat. Cook for 5-10 minutes, until bubbling. Slightly smash some of the blueberries with the back of a fork.
2. In a small bowl, stir together the arrowroot powder and 1 Tbs. of water. Remove the saucepan of berries from the heat. While stirring constantly, add the arrowroot mixture into the blueberry mixture. Let cool until no longer hot and serve. The sauce with become even thicker when chilled.

**You can store the sauce in the fridge for a few days.

221. Fluffy Coconut Flour Waffles

Ingredients
8 free-range organic eggs
1/2 cup melted butter or ghee (organic and preferably grass-fed)
1/2 cup coconut flour
1/4 teaspoon low sodium salt
1/4 teaspoon baking soda
1/4 cup canned coconut milk
1 tsp stevia drops
Instructions:
1. Take out your waffle maker.
2. In a large bowl add the eggs and beat with an electric hand mixer for 30 seconds until the eggs are well beaten.
3. Add the melted butter or ghee slowly into the eggs while you are still mixing.
4. Add the coconut flour, pink salt, baking soda and coconut milk.
5. Mix with the hand mixer for 45 second on low until the batter becomes thicker.
6. Heat up your waffle maker and make the waffles according to your maker's specifications..
7. Serve with butter or ghee, mashed strawberries (recipe here) or fresh maple syrup

222. Sexy Savory Pannukakku

Ingredients
1/4 cup coconut oil
1/4 cup coconut flour
1/4 cup arrowroot powder
1/4 teaspoon low sodium salt
1 cup light coconut milk (canned)
8 eggs
2 teaspoons pure vanilla extract
1 tsp stevia
Instructions
1. Preheat the oven to 400 degrees. Place the butter in a 9 by 13 inch baking pan and place it in the oven to let it melt.
2. In a medium mixing bowl, stir together the coconut flour, arrowroot, and salt. Whisk in the coconut milk until there are no lumps of starch. Whisk in the eggs, vanilla, and stevia.
3. Remove the hot pan from the oven and pour the batter onto the hot butter (pour slowly to avoid splatters of hot butter). Return the pan to the hot oven and bake for 15-20 minutes, or until the edges has puffed up and the center is set. Serve right away, topped with warmed berries, if desired.

223. Fudgy Coconut Flour Brownies

Ingredients
1/2 cup minus 1 Tbs. coconut
1/2 cup cocoa powder
1/2 cup plus 2 Tbs. coconut oil, melted
3 eggs, at room temperature
1/2 cup almond milk
2 Tsp stevia
1 tsp. vanilla extract, optional

Instructions
1. Preheat the oven to 300 and grease a glass baking dish (8x8 or 9x9).
2. Mix together all ingredients. You can do this by hand or with an electric mixer or high-powered blender.
3. Pour into the baking dish and bake for 30-35 minutes, until a toothpick inserted into the center comes out clean. Cool for 30 minutes before cutting or removing from the pan.
4. These store well at room temperature or in the fridge for a few days. Make sure you keep them in an airtight container.

224. Delectable Pumpkin Bars

Ingredients:
15 oz. pumpkin puree (about 1 1/2 cups)
3/4 cup coconut flour
3/4 cup almond milk
1 1/2 teaspoons ground cinnamon
3/4 teaspoon ground ginger
1/4 teaspoon ground cloves
3/4 teaspoon baking soda
1/4 teaspoon low sodium salt
2 large eggs

Instruction
1. Preheat the oven to 350F and grease a 9"x9" baking dish well with coconut oil. Combine all of the ingredients in a large mixing bowl, and stir well until no clumps remain. Transfer the batter to the greased baking dish, and use a spatula to smooth the top.
2. Bake at 350F for 40-45 minutes, or until the edges are golden and the center is firm.
3. Allow to cool completely, then cut into squares and serve. Store in in the fridge for up to a week. (They're delicious straight out of the fridge, too!)

225. Mouthwatering Lemon Bars

Ingredients:
Crust:
2 cups Sifted Coconut Flour
½ teaspoon low sodium Salt
½ cup almond milk
1tsp stevia
16 tablespoons Room Temperature Virgin Coconut Oil {= 1 cup}

Filling:
1 ½ cup Fresh Lemon Juice
1 cup almond milk
½ cup coconut oil
1 tsp stevia
2 tablespoons Lemon Zest
8 Eggs

Instructions:
Crust:
1. Preheat oven to 350 F.
2. Line a 9×13 inch baking dish with parchment paper.
3. Whisk the coconut flour with salt.
4. Thoroughly stir in the milk and coconut oil until it's evenly mixed and crumbly.
5. Add the room-temperature coconut oil and stir until it's evenly combined.
6. Pat the dough down into the bottom of the baking dish for an even thickness.
7. Bake at 350 for approximately 17 minutes or until it starts to brown.
8. Remove from the oven and let cool on the counter while you prepare the filling.

FILLING:
1. Mix stevia with the lemon juice.
2. Working quickly, whisk in the eggs.
3. Whisk in the lemon zest.
4. Pour the filling into the now cooled crust.
5. Bake at 350 for 25 – 30 minutes or until it's stiffened.
6. Let it cool on the counter for 30 minutes than the refrigerator for 3 hours or overnight.
7. Cut into squares and serve chilled.

226. Yummy Pumpkin Bars

Ingredients
1/2 cup coconut manna
1/2 cup coconut oil
1/4 heaping cup coconut flour
1 1/2 cup cooked winter squash (butternut or pumpkin)
A pinch of low sodium salt
2 tsp. cinnamon
1 tsp. ginger
1/4 cup almond milk
1 tsp stevia

Instructions
1. On the stove, gently melt coconut oil and manna until melted.
2. In food processor, add squash, spices, coconut flour, salt, milk and stevia. Pour melted coconut oil and manna on top and blend for 30 seconds being sure all the big pieces of squash are blended.
3. Line a square 8x8 brownie pan with parchment paper. Scoop the bar filling into the pan and use a spatula to smooth it out. Bake for 25 min at 350 degrees. Remove from oven, let cool, cover and put in fridge until completely chilled; about 3 hours.

227. Delicious Coconut Biscuits

Ingredients
4 large eggs, yolks and whites divided
1/2 cup coconut flour
1/4 teaspoon baking soda
1/2 teaspoon cream of tartar
1/2 teaspoon low sodium salt
4 tablespoons coconut oil, room temperature
1 tsp stevia

Instructions
1. Preheat oven to 400 degrees.
2. In a medium bowl, whisk the egg whites until frothy and at least doubled in size. Mix in the yolks until no streaks remain then add stevia.
3. In a separate bowl, combine the flour, baking soda, cream of tartar and salt.
4. Using a fork or pastry cutter, mix the butter into the dry ingredients until you have pea-sized bits of butter.
5. Fold the flour mixture into the egg mixture, incorporating well (the batter will be rather wet, but the coconut flour will start to absorb some of the liquid. Do not add more coconut flour!).
6. Using a 1/4 cup measuring cup, scoop the batter onto a parchment lined baking sheet.
7. Bake for 15-20 minutes or until golden brown and a toothpick inserted into the biscuit comes out clean.

228. Beautiful Butternut Pitta Surprise

Ingredients
- 1 Tbs. coconut flour
- 1 1/2 tsp. grass fed gelatin
- 3 Tbs. well-cooked and mashed butternut squash (or sweet potato)
- 1 Tbs. coconut oil
- 1 egg
- Low sodium salt (to taste)
- **(You can double the recipe if desired)

Instructions
1. Prepare all the ingredients and have them at room temperature.
2. Preheat the oven to 400 and line a baking sheet with parchment paper. Stir together the coconut flour and gelatin.
3. Stir together the squash and the coconut oil until smooth. Stir in the coconut flour/gelatin mixture until combined, and then stir in the egg and salt.
4. Spoon into rounds on the baking sheet. Make sure that you spoon out the same sizes. It's up to you but I prefer a bit thicker.
5. Bake for about 12 minutes, and then carefully peel them off the parchment paper and flip. Bake for another 5 minutes (or longer), until they are dry to the touch and pliable. (They will take longer to cook if they are thicker and they will cook faster if they are thinner.)
6. Let cool completely, then enjoy within an hour or so of baking for the best texture.

229. Onion Herb Coconut Biscuits

Ingredients
6 Tbsp. coconut flour
6 Tbsp. coconut oil, melted
2 eggs
1/4 cup very finely minced onion
2 garlic cloves, finely minced
2 Tbs. GAPS/SCD yogurt or additive free coconut milk
1 Tbs. fresh chopped herbs (parsley, dill, thyme... whatever you have) OR 3/4 tsp. dried herbs
1/4 tsp. baking soda
1/2 tsp. apple cider vinegar

Instructions
1. Preheat the oven to 350. Line two baking sheets with parchment paper.
2. Mix together the coconut flour, oil, eggs, onion, garlic, yogurt/coconut milk, and herbs Let sit for 5 minutes; the batter will thicken slightly.
3. Mix in the baking soda and vinegar. Drop a spoonful of batter onto the baking sheets. Use the back of a spoon to spread the batter into circles about 1/2" thick. The batter will not spread very much when baking.
4. Bake for 12-15 minutes, until moist but cooked through. Cool at least 10 minutes before serving, or they will be too crumbly.

230. Oniony Delishy Biscuits

Ingredients
1/3 cut coconut flour
¼ cup coconut flour, melted
4 eggs
1/4 tsp low sodium salt
1/4 tsp cream of tartar
1/8 tsp baking soda
1 cup shredded onion

Instruction
1. Preheat oven to 400 degrees
2. Put flour, salt, cream of tartar and baking soda in a small bowl
3. Put eggs and coconut oil in a mixing bowl, and whisk until smooth
4. Add flour mixture, and whisk until no lumps remain
5. Stir in the onion
6. Drop by spoonful onto lightly oiled baking sheet
7. Bake 8-10 minutes until lightly browned
8. Remove from baking sheet

231. Crisp Coconut Flour Tortillas

Ingredients
1/2 cup coconut flour
1/2 teaspoon grain free baking powder
1/4 teaspoon low sodium salt
1 1/2 cup egg whites (or 16 egg whites)*
3/4 cup almond milk

Instruction
1. Mix all of the ingredients in a non-reactive bowl.
2. Let it sit for 10 minutes so the coconut flour can soak up some of the moisture, and then whisk again. The batter should be runnier than that of pancakes, about the same as a crepe batter.
3. Heat a non-stick skillet over medium high heat and spray with oil or melt enough butter to coat the bottom and sides of pan.
4. Pour 1/4 cup of the batter into the pan, swirling the pan while you pour to ensure the bottom is coated and the tortilla is thin.
5. Once the bottom looks set (about 1 minute), carefully release the sides of the tortilla with a rubber spatula and turn over. Alternatively, you could use a frittata pan, or turn the tortilla into another hot and greased pan or greased griddle. This may help the tortilla to stay in one piece. If your first couple breaks, don't fret and don't throw them away. Add a little more coconut flour and try again, but keep the broken ones to use as filling if you're making enchiladas.
6. Spray the pan again, and repeat above steps until all the batter is used. Layer the tortillas on a plate and set aside until you're read to fill them and bake.

232. Easy Delish Pizza Crust Recipe

Ingredients
1 cup tapioca flour (starch) (plus more for rolling out dough)
1/3 cup + 2-3 tablespoons coconut flour, separated
1 teaspoon low sodium salt
1/2 cup olive oil
1/2 cup warm water
1 large egg, whisked

Instructions
1. Preheat oven to 450 degrees F
2. Combine the tapioca flour (you can substitute arrowroot flour/starch), salt and 1/3 cup coconut flour in a medium bowl.
3. Pour in oil and warm water and stir. Your mixture will look something like this.
4. Add the whisked egg and continue mixing until well combined.
5. Add two to three more tablespoons of coconut flour – one tablespoon at a time – until the mixture is soft but somewhat sticky dough.
6. Turn out the dough onto a surface sprinkled with tapioca flour and knead it gently until it is in a manageable ball that does not stick to your hands.
7. Place the pizza dough ball onto a sheet of parchment paper. Use a tapioca floured rolling pin to carefully roll out the dough until it is fairly thin. You may end up using another few tablespoons of tapioca at this point. You will need it to keep the dough from being too sticky. But don't overwork the dough or add TOO much more tapioca or your dough will be too dense.
8. Place the rolled out dough (on its parchment paper) into the preheated oven onto a hot pizza stone or sheet pan. I used a pizza stone that was left in the oven while it was heating up. You may have different results if you put it on a sheet pan or with the paper directly on the oven rack.
9. Bake for 12-15 minutes depending on how "done" the crust should be before putting on toppings. Here's what it looked like after 12 minutes on the pizza stone.

233. Coconut Pretty Pizza Crust

Ingredients
1 egg
1 tablespoon cream of buckwheat
1 tablespoon coconut flour
1/8 teaspoon baking soda

Instructions
Preheat oven to 425.
1. Mix all ingredients in a bowl until well combined.
2. Line a cookie tray with parchment paper and spread the cheese mixture on the paper as thinly as possible, using the back of a spoon or fork.
3. Reduce heat to 400 and bake on the top rack for about 15 minutes, or until the crust is starting to look golden in places. Remove from the oven and add desired toppings.
4. You can store this in the fridge for up to 3 days.

234. Creamy Appetizing Croissant

Ingredients
3 eggs, separated.
¼ tsp cream of tartar, where to buy this
2 tbsp organic coconut cream, softened.
2 tbsp coconut oil, melted
2 tbsp coconut flour
15 drops liquid stevia
½ tsp baking soda + ¼ tsp cream of tartar, mix together in separate pinch bowl.
⅛ tsp low sodium salt

Kitchen Tools:
2 large mixing bowls
1 donut pan, or bagel pan
1 electric hand mixer or stand mixer
1 pinch bowl (small bowl)

Instructions
1. Preheat oven to 300 F, and grease or oil a bagel or donut pan (even if it's a non- stick type).
2. Separate egg whites from yolks, and place whites in one mixing bowl, and yolks in another mixing bowl.
3. Add cream of tartar to egg whites and whip with stand mixer or hand mixer until stiff peaks form. Set aside.
4. Beat egg yolks in separate mixing bowl and add: creamed coconut, melted coconut oil, coconut flour, stevia, baking soda and cream of tartar mixture, and sea salt. Beat egg yolk mixture until thoroughly combined.
5. Gently fold egg yolk mixture into egg white mixture until combined (careful not to stir or beat (should still be a whipped meringue texture).
6. Spoon mixture into bagel pan, and spread around, with the back of a spoon, in the pan forms. Wipe off excess that gets on the bagel hole with a damp paper towel.
7. Bake for 20 to 25 minutes or until tops and edges are slightly browning. Should check at 20 minutes, as all oven temperatures can vary.
8. Remove and cool. Use a butter knife in between the pan and the croissant, and slide around to loosen from pan.
Store unused portions in a covered container or zipper bag, put it in the fridge. Bagels can be reheated.

235. Delicious Gnocchi Balls

Ingredients
3 eggs, beaten
4 tbsp coconut flour
1 tsp garlic powder
1/4 tsp low sodium salt

Instructions
1. Mix the coconut flour and beaten eggs well.
2. Add the garlic powder and salt and mix well into dough.
3. Place the dough on a sheet of cling film and roll into a long sausage shape.
4. Wrap up with the cling film and place in the refrigerator. Chill the dough for a minimum of 30 minutes.
5. Bring a saucepan of water to the boil.
6. Remove the Gnocchi dough from the refrigerator and cut into small bite sized pieces.
7. Place the pieces into the boiling water, reduce the heat to medium and cook for 4-5 minutes. Remove with a slotted spoon. Repeat until all gnocchi are cooked.
8. Top with the sauce of your choice.

*Makes about 8-10 gnocchi.

236. Crispy Coconut Crackers

Ingredients
4 ounces shredded coconut
4 tablespoons butter (2 ounces or 1/2 stick), softened
1/4 cup tapioca flour
1 tablespoon coconut flour
1/2 teaspoon baking soda
1/4 teaspoon powdered mustard
1/4 teaspoon powdered onion

Instructions:
1. Preheat your oven to 350F. Line a baking sheet with parchment paper or a silicone mat.
2. Combine all ingredients in a food processor. Buzz until a ball of dough has formed.
3. Use your hands to shape dough into 1-inch balls. Place balls on the baking sheet, leaving about 3 inches of space between each.
4. Bake until the edges are slightly browned, about 10 minutes.

237. Tempting Custard Pie

Ingredients
4 eggs 2 cups coconut milk
1/4 cup expeller-pressed coconut oil (softened works best)
1/2 cup almond milk
1 tsp stevia
1/2 cup coconut flour
1/2 teaspoon baking powder
1/2 teaspoon low sodium salt
1 tablespoon vanilla (or 2 vanilla beans scraped)
1 cup shredded dried coconut

Instructions
1. Preheat oven to 325 degrees ºF.
2. Place all ingredients into a blender and blend for about 10 seconds (or until thoroughly mixed)
3. Pour into a pie dish greased with coconut oil.
4. Bake for 55 minutes in preheated oven. Serve warm (or cold the next day for breakfast!)

* For the freshest coconut milk make homemade coconut milk.

238. Nutritious Paleo Tortillas

Ingredients
1/4 cup coconut flour (40 g)
1/4 teaspoon baking powder
8 egg whites (240 g or 1 cup)
1/2 cup water
A pinch of low sodium salt
coconut oil (as needed, for greasing the press or pan)
Instructions
1. In a bowl mix all ingredients. Set aside for five minutes. The batter takes about that long to hydrate and thicken.
*If necessary grease your tortilla press or pan with coconut oil.
Make the tortillas:
1. In a preheated electric tortilla press: Pour about a little less than 1/4 cup of batter onto the tortilla press. Quickly smooth out using a heat resistant spoon, and press the top of the press down to distribute the rest of the batter. Cook until the indicator on the press goes off.
2. In a pan over medium heat: Pour a little less than 1/4 cup of batter onto the pan. Quickly smooth out using a heat resistant spoon. Cook for 1 to 2 minutes or until the edges of the tortilla start to turn golden brown. Then flip and cook for an additional minute or two.
3. Transfer tortillas to a plate and cover with a paper towel to keep warm.
4. Serve with desired toppings and do your best to keep away from within hungry doggy mouths.

239. Luscious Chocolate-Caramel Brownies

Ingredients
1/4 cup coconut flour
1 1/4 cup cacao powder
4 eggs
1 teaspoon low sodium salt
1 teaspoon baking soda
1/2 cup almond milk
1 ½ tsp stevia
1 tablespoon vanilla extract
1/3 cup coconut oil
1/3 cup dark chocolate chips
1 homemade caramel recipe

Instructions:
1. Preheat oven to 350 degrees Fahrenheit.
2. Mix dry ingredients in one bowl and wet ingredients in a second bowl.
3. Combine both mixtures and stir until all ingredients are incorporated together.
4. Pour the mixture into a greased 8x8 pan.
5. Top with chocolate chips and/or nuts if desired, and bake for 25–30 minutes.
6. Let cool and then drizzle with caramel sauce.

240. Fudgy Pumpkin Blondies

Ingredients
2 cups blanched almond flour
½ cup flaxseed meal
2 teaspoons ground cinnamon (optional)
½ cup raw coconut palm sugar
½ teaspoon salt
1 egg
1 cup pumpkin puree
1 tablespoon vanilla extract
⅓ cup (or more) chocolate chunks

Instructions
mix together the almond flour, flaxseed meal, cinnamon, coconut palm sugar, chocolate chunks and salt
in a separate bowl, whisk the egg, pumpkin and vanilla extract
using a rubber spatula, gently mix dry and wet ingredients to form a batter being careful not to over mix or the batter will get oily and dense
spoon the batter onto a 9-inch pan lined with parchment paper
bake at 350°F until a toothpick inserted into the centre comes out clean, approximately 25 minutes

241. Spinach Brownies Revisited

Ingredients:
1 ¼ cups frozen chopped spinach (measured frozen)
1 cup pureed green plantain (1 large plantain or 1 1/2 medium plantains)
6 oz semisweet chocolate (substitute bittersweet for a less sweet brownie)
½ cup extra virgin coconut oil
½ cup palm shortening (or substitute butter)
6 eggs
1 Tbsp honey
1 Tbsp molasses
½ cup cocoa powder
1 Tbsp vanilla (or substitute espresso)
¼ tsp baking soda
½ tsp salt
½ tsp cream of tartar
pinch cinnamon

Instructions:
Preheat oven to 325F. Line a 9"x13" baking pan with wax paper or use a silicone baking pan.
Melt coconut oil and chocolate together over low heat on the stove top or medium power in the microwave. Add vanilla and stir to incorporate. Let cool.
Mix cocoa powder, baking soda, cream of tartar, salt and cinnamon.
Blend spinach, plantain, egg, honey and molasses together in a food processor or blender, until completely smooth (2-4 minutes).
Add palm shortening to food processor and process until full incorporated.
Add melted chocolate mixture to egg mixture slowly and processing/blending constantly.
Mix in dry ingredients and process/stir to fully incorporate.
Pour batter into prepared baking pan and spread out with a spatula.
Bake for 40 minutes. Cool completely in pan. Cut into squares. Enjoy!

Paleo Diet Recipes 365 Days of Paleo and Coconut Recipes by Mercedes Del Rey

242. Celebratory Chocolate Hazelnut Cupcakes

Ingredients:

2 large (or 3 medium) zucchini, grated (about 3 cups grated)
4 eggs
2 cups Hazelnuts
5 drops stevia liquid (May need a few more – please taste test)
1/4 cup coconut oil (room temperature)
1/3 cup Tapioca Flour (this is the same thing as Tapioca Starch)
1 cup cocoa powder
1 Tsp Vanilla Extract
1 tsp Baking Soda
½ tsp low sodium Salt

Instructions

Preheat oven to 350F. Line a muffin pan with paper liners, use Silicone Muffin Cups. or bake in a silicone muffin pan.
Grind hazelnuts in a Food Processor or Magic Bullet until they are super fine and almost turning into hazelnut butter.
Finely grate zucchini (you could even process in a food processor).
Combine ground hazelnuts, grated zucchini and the rest of the ingredients together in a bowl. The batter is quite runny. That's okay–that's why these cupcakes are so fudgy.
As an alternative you can combine all ingredients in a food processor or blender and process/blend until smooth.
Pour mixture into prepared muffin pan and bake for 30 minutes.
Let cool completely before icing or serving. Enjoy!

Paleo Diet Recipes 365 Days of Paleo and Coconut Recipes by Mercedes Del Rey

243. Bursting Banana Cupcakes (nut-free) with Whipped White Chocolate Sesame Frosting

Ingredients (frosting):
3 oz cocoa butter
1 Madagascar vanilla bean
5 drops stevia liquid (May need a few more – please taste test)
1/4 cup tahini (aka sesame seed butter)
1 tsp arrowroot powder
1/4 `room temperature coconut oil

Instructions
Melt cocoa butter (you can do this in a double boiler or in the microwave). Add stevia to melted cocoa butter and whisk until cane juice has dissolved.
Cut the vanilla bean lengthwise and scrape out the vanilla seeds with a sharp knife (save the pod for making vanilla ice cream or some other dish where you simmer the vanilla pod in coconut milk). Add to cocoa butter.
Add the remaining ingredients and whisk together until fully combined.
Allow to cool to room temperature (because of the high melting point of cocoa butter, this takes a long long time—if you want to speed it up, put it in the fridge and whisk aggressively every 5 minutes while it cools). Whisk every so often (maybe every half hour) just to make sure it doesn't separate or clump up.
Whip aggressively by hand (or you could use a hand mixer or blender) and generously frost your cupcakes!

Ingredients (cupcakes):
3 large (or 4 medium) overripe bananas
3 eggs
3 Tbsp extra virgin coconut oil
5 drops stevia liquid (May need a few more – please taste test)
1 tsp vanilla
1/3 cup coconut flour
1/3 cup arrowroot powder
1 tsp baking soda
1/8 tsp low sodium salt

Instructions
Preheat oven to 350F.
Grease a muffin pan or put paper liners. I actually use a silicone muffin pan just because it's so easy and ends up saving me tons of time!
Combine all of the ingredients in a blender or food processor (yes, it really is that easy). Blend or process about 1-2 minutes until you have a thick and smooth batter.
Pour batter into prepared muffin pan. You can make your cupcakes a bit bigger by dividing into 10 muffin cups or a bit smaller by dividing into 12 muffin cups.
Bake for 40 minutes (45 if you only make 10). Remove from oven and let cool completely before frosting. Enjoy!

244. Lovely Lemon Cupcakes with Lemon Frosting (2 Variations)(Nut-Free)

Ingredients (Lemon Caramel Frosting):

5 drops stevia liquid (May need a few more – please taste test)
2/3 cup fresh Lemon Juice
¼ tsp Baking Soda
½ room temperature coconut oil

Instructions
1. Heat stevia and lemon juice in a medium-sized saucepot over low heat. Reduce to 1 cup volume, being very careful not to let it burn (this will take 10-15 minutes).
2. Remove from heat and immediately stir in baking soda. It will froth and expand. Stir vigorously for 15-20 seconds, then pour into a bowl and let cool to room temperature.
3. Mix in coconut oil until completely combined.
4. Store in an airtight container at room temperature for several days or store in the fridge for longer-term storage (warm up to room temperature before frosting cupcakes).

Ingredients (Lemon Coconut Butter Frosting):
½ cup Coconut Cream Concentrate (a.k.a. Coconut Butter or Creamed Coconut)
¼ cup fresh Lemon Juice
5 drops stevia liquid (May need a few more – please taste test)
1. If you are opening a new bottle or box of coconut cream concentrate and the oil has separated out, heat the jar (or remove the contents of the box to a glass jar) by placing it a pot or bowl and surrounding with hot water. Let it sit until it's warmed enough to stir thoroughly. Let cool to room temperature.
2. Mix coconut cream concentrate, lemon juice and stevia until thoroughly combined.
3. Store in an airtight container at room temperature for several days or store in the fridge for longer-term storage (warm up to room temperature before frosting cupcakes).

Ingredients (Lemon Cupcakes):
½ cup Coconut Flour
¼ cup Tapioca Flour
½ tsp Baking Soda
6 Eggs
5 drops stevia liquid (May need a few more – please taste test)
¼ cup fresh Lemon Juice (roughly juice of two lemons)
2 Tbsp finely grated Lemon Zest (roughly zest from two lemons)
Instructions
1. Preheat oven to 350F. Line a muffin tin with paper muffin cup liners.
2. Blend all ingredients together in a a until a smooth batter forms. Let the batter rest for 2-3 minutes to thicken.
3. Pour batter into prepared muffin tin. Each cup should be filled approximately ¾ full (or slightly more).
4. Bake for 22-23 minutes, until starting to turn golden brown along the edges (should pass a toothpick test).
5. Carefully remove cupcakes from pan and cool on a wire rack. Let cupcakes cool completely before frosting.
6. Spread a generous amount of frosting (which ever you chose) on each cupcake. Candied lemon zest and edible flowers make great decorations for these cupcakes.
7. Enjoy!

Paleo Diet Recipes 365 Days of Paleo and Coconut Recipes by Mercedes Del Rey

245. Sexy Red Velvet Chocolate Cupcakes With Coconut-Cherry Glaze

Ingredients
¼ cup beets, peeled and finely grated
1¼ cup blanched almond flour
½ teaspoon baking soda
2 tablespoons raw cacao powder
¼ cup coconut oil, melted
7 tablespoons coconut milk, full fat
1 teaspoon vanilla extract
1 teaspoon apple cider vinegar
2 tablespoons raw stevia (add more if you like it sweeter)
1 egg
¼ cup chocolate chips

Coconut-cherry Glaze:
1 can (13.5 ounces) coconut milk, full fat
1 teaspoon vanilla extract
6 fresh cherries, pitted

Instructions
Preheat the oven to 350°F and line a muffin tin with baking cups.
Mix together the blanched almond flour, baking soda and raw cacao powder.
In a separate bowl, whisk together the coconut oil, coconut milk, vanilla extract, apple cider vinegar, stevia, egg and grated beets.
Using a rubber spatula, gently mix the wet and dry ingredients together.
Fold chocolate chips into the batter.
Spoon batter into prepared muffin tin, filling each to the top.
Bake until a toothpick inserted into the center comes out clean, about 30-35 minutes.
Set pan on a wire rack to cool, then top with the coconut glaze and a fresh cherry.
Coconut Glaze:
Place a can of full fat coconut milk in the fridge overnight.
Scoop the coconut cream that forms on top of the can into a bowl, being careful not to mix with the water in the bottom of the can.
Add the vanilla extract and using a handheld or stand electrical mixer, whip the coconut cream until fluffy.

246. Party Pink Velvet Cupcakes with Vanilla Frosting

Ingredients
Cupcakes
1/2 cup coconut oil, melted
5 drops stevia liquid (May need a few more – please taste test)
3 eggs
1 teaspoon vanilla extract
3/4 cup tapioca flour
1/2 cup coconut flour
1 teaspoon baking powder
2 tablespoons beet powder (works without it)
pinch of low sodium salt

Frosting
1/2 cup room temperature coconut oil
5 drops stevia liquid (May need a few more – please taste test)
1 teaspoon vanilla extract
2 tablespoons tapioca flour or arrowroot powder
2 teaspoons coconut flour
1 tablespoon chilled coconut milk fat (thick stuff from top of can)

Instructions
Cupcakes
Preheat oven to 350 degrees Fahrenheit
In a stand mixer or large bowl, mix together coconut oil, stevia, eggs and vanilla extract with a mixer or whisk
In a separate bowl, whisk tapioca flour, coconut flour, baking powder, beet powder and salt together
Slowly mix the dry mixture in with the wet mixture, adding ¼ cup at a time until well mixed
Scoop your batter into muffin liners in a muffin pan. Fill each well 2/3 of the way and you should get 10 cupcakes
Place in oven and bake for 18-20 minutes or until cooked through. Use a toothpick to poke through a muffin to make sure the toothpick comes out clean
Frosting
Combine the coconut oil shortening, stevia, vanilla, tapioca flour and coconut flour in the bowl of a stand mixer with a whisk attachment or a large mixing bowl
Using the stand mixer or a hand mixer, beat until smooth
Add your chilled coconut milk and beat until well combined. Do not over mix or your frosting might separate
Once your cupcakes are completely cool, use immediately by placing in a piping bag or ziploc bag with a corner cut off to frost your cupcakes

247. Chocolate Cupcakes with Coconut Cream Filling

Ingredients
Cupcakes
1/4 cup coconut flour
1/4 cup organic cocoa powder
4 large eggs (at room temperature)
1/4 cup coconut oil
5 drops stevia liquid (May need a few more – please taste test)
1/4 tsp baking soda
1 tsp lemon juice
Pinch of low sodium salt
Cream Filling (Optional)
Cream from 1 13.5 oz can of full fat coconut milk (refrigerate the can overnight and scoop out the cream that rises to the top)
5 drops stevia liquid (May need a few more – please taste test)
1 tsp vanilla extract
Chocolate Frosting
3 very ripe avocados
1/2 cup organic cocoa powder
5 drops stevia liquid (May need a few more – please taste test)
2 Tbsp grass fed butter or coconut oil, melted

Instructions
Preheat oven to 350 F
Combine the coconut flour, cocoa powder, sweetener, baking soda, and low sodium salt.
In a separate bowl, combine the eggs, coconut oil, and lemon juice.
Add the dry ingredients to the wet and mix to combine.
Line a muffin tin with 7 cupcake liners.
Fill cupcake liners evenly with the batter and bake for 18 - 20 minutes or until cooked through.
Allow to cool before filling with cream and topping with the icing.
Once cool, cut a small whole in the middle of each cupcake, reserving the lid/top of the hole that was cut out.
Fill with cream (directions below) and place the lid/top back on the cupcake to cover the hole.
Pipe chocolate frosting (directions below) onto each cupcake and serve.
For the cream filling
Combine the coconut cream, sweetener, and vanilla and mix until smooth. Pipe the cream into the hole cut out of the cupcake.
For the chocolate frosting
Place the meat of the avocados in a mixer and mix until completely smooth.
Add the cocoa powder and sweetener and mix until thoroughly incorporated.
Add the butter and mix to combine.

248. Delish Apple Pie Cupcakes with Cinnamon Frosting

Ingredients:
WET INGREDIENTS
5 Eggs, room temperature
1/2 cup applesauce (you can make your own or use a sugar-free pre-made brand)
5 drops stevia liquid (May need a few more – please taste test)
1/3 cup coconut oil, melted

DRY INGREDIENTS
1/4 cup finely ground blanch almond flour
1/2 cup coconut flour
1/2 tsp. low sodium salt
1/2 tsp. baking powder

FROSTING INGREDIENTS:
1 cup coconut oil
3 drops stevia liquid
2 tsp. cinnamon
Dash low sodium salt

Instructions
1. Preheat oven to 350F. Line muffin pan with baking cups.
2. Combine all wet ingredients in a medium sized mixing bowl. Beat on medium with a hand mixer for about 30 seconds.
3. Combine all dry ingredients in another medium sized bowl. Mix together with a fork to break apart any clumps.
4. Add the dry ingredients to the wet ingredients and beat for about 20 seconds. Make sure all ingredients are combined.
5. Fill each lined muffin tin about 3/4 of the way full. Bake for 25-30 minutes or until a toothpick comes out clean in the center.
6. Take the cupcakes out of the oven and set aside to cool completely. All the way cooled! But feel free to sneak one to nibble on while the rest cool off.
7. Once the cupcakes have cooled, make the frosting! Combine all of the ingredients into a medium mixing bowl and beat on medium speed for about 30 seconds until well combines. Ice those cupcakes and get to eating!

Paleo Diet Recipes 365 Days of Paleo and Coconut Recipes by Mercedes Del Rey

249. Pumpkin Coco Cupcakes with creamy cinnamon filling

Makes 12 cupcakes
Cupcake:
1 cup pumpkin puree
3 eggs
5 drops stevia liquid (May need a few more – please taste test)
1 Tbs raw apple cider vinegar
2 Tbs melted butter or coconut oil
1 tsp vanilla extract
1 ½ cups almond flour
2 Tbs coconut flour
2 tsp cinnamon
½ tsp cardamom powder
1/2 tsp ginger powder
¼ tsp each nutmeg, allspice and cloves
¾ tsp sea low sodium salt
¾ tsp baking soda
2 oz unsweetened baking chocolate (can also use chocolate chips)

Instructions
Preheat oven to 350 F. Line a cupcake pan with liners.
In a medium bowl, whisk together the pumpkin puree, eggs, stevia, butter and vanilla extract. Mix until smooth. Add in the flours, spices, low sodium salt and baking soda and stir until well combined. Add the vinegar.
Using a sharp knife, cut the baking chocolate into small chunks. Fold into the cupcake batter to evenly distribute.
Portion out into lined cupcake tins, until they are almost completely full of batter; these will not rise very much, so no need to worry too much about them getting too big.
Bake for 25 minutes. Check with a toothpick to make sure they are done; if the toothpick comes out clean, they are ready. If not, add 5 more minutes to the baking time.
Let cool completely before frosting.

Frosting:
8 oz. Full fat organic creamed coconut
¼ cup coconut butter, softened
5 drops stevia liquid (May need a few more – please taste test)
1 tsp vanilla extract
1 ½ Tbs cinnamon

Using a strong fork, cream together the cream and butter until smooth. Stir in the stevia, vanilla and cinnamon, and stir well until creamy and well combined.
Use a piping bag or simply a knife to top the cooled cupcakes with the buttercream frosting.

250. Bursting Banana Choco Cupcakes

Ingredients:
2 cups almond meal
1/2 cup almond butter
2 ripe bananas
1/4 cup cocoa powder, unsweetened of course
1/2 cup coconut palm sugar
1/2 cup chocolate chips (I like Enjoy Life brand)
2 eggs
1 tsp pure organic vanilla extract
1 tsp low sodium salt
1/2 tsp baking soda
1 tsp apple cider vinegar
paper muffin liners

Instructions
1. Instead of mixing wet and dry ingredients separate from each other, I just built it all in one bowl. Any opportunity I get to save myself from having more dishes to do, you bet I will take!
2. Preheat the oven to 350 degrees. Mash the bananas, mix in the almond butter and coconut palm sugar, add the vanilla extract, salt, eggs, baking soda and vinegar. Make it chocolaty and dump in the cocoa powder. Mix that in good and start adding the almond meal a cup at a time to make sure it all incorporates well. When a nice batter forms, make it even chocolatier and dump in the half cup of chocolate chips.
3. Line a muffin pan with the paper liners, fill each cup with batter. You'll get a dozen.
4. Bake for 20 minutes and let cool before eating. The tops get a brownie-like crust, the cake is moist and light.

251. Jam and 'Cream' Cupcakes

cupcakes
1/2 cup coconut flour, sifted
1/4 cup arrowroot (tapioca flour), sifted
4 eggs
5 drops stevia liquid (May need a few more – please taste test)
3 tablespoons coconut oil
1 cup full fat coconut cream
1/2 teaspoon concentrated natural vanilla extract
pinch of low sodium salt
1 teaspoon baking powder
sugar free strawberry jam*
1 punnet of strawberries (250 grams or approximately 1 heaped cup of chopped strawberries)
2 tablespoons chia seeds
2 drops stevia
Place the ingredients into blender or food processor and blend until smooth and well combined. Pour / spoon the mixture into a container and place in the fridge to thicken.
'cream'*
1 cup raw macadamias
1/2 teaspoon concentrated natural vanilla extract
pinch of low sodium salt

Instructions
1. Place the ingredients into your blender or food processor and blend at high speed until you have a lovely, smooth macadamia butter. I leave this at room temperature as I find it easier to work with when assembling the cupcakes. After that I store the remaining butter in the fridge.
2. Preheat your oven to 175 degrees Celsius or 350 degrees Fahrenheit.
3. Line nine holes of a standard muffin tray with cupcake cases.
4. In a medium sized bowl beat together your stevia and coconut oil. Add in the eggs, coconut cream and vanilla. 5. Add the flours and when smooth and well combined gently add the salt and baking powder.
6. Spoon the mixture evenly into your nine cases.
7. Bake for 25 minutes.
8. Allow to cool slightly before moving from the tray to a cooling rack.
9. Leave the cakes to cool completely before using a small, sharp knife to remove the tops of the cupcakes and create a small indent in the cake. Fill the cake with a teaspoon of jam and a teaspoon of 'cream' (macadamia butter).
10. Gently place the cupcake 'lid' back on top.
11. Eat and enjoy!!!

252. Delicious Yellow Cupcake Recipe

Ingredients
Cake
½ cup of sifted Organic coconut flour
5 large eggs
⅓ cup of butter or ghee or coconut oil
1 teaspoon vanilla
5 drops stevia liquid (May need a few more – please taste test)
1 cup of applesauce
1 teaspoon baking powder
1 teaspoon baking soda

Instructions:
Combine the coconut flour, baking powder and baking soda in a bowl and blend.
Add in all the liquid ingredients; mix well with a spoon.
Pour into the cupcake tins and bake at 350 degrees for 20 minutes.
Frost and enjoy!

253. Perfect Pear & Nutmeg Cupcakes

Ingredients
2 ripe pears, peeled, de-cored and chopped into small pieces
1 tsp nutmeg
1 tbsp water
1/4 cup coconut flour
2 large eggs
1/4 cup coconut oil or melted butter
5 drops stevia liquid (May need a few more – please taste test)
1/4 tsp baking powder

Instructions
Add the pear, water, 5 drops stevia and 1/2 tsp of nutmeg to a saucepan. Let the mixture simmer over a medium heat until the pears soften (about 15 mins). Either mash with a hand-masher or transfer to a blender and puree. Set aside to cool.
Sieve the coconut flour, the remaining tsp of nutmeg and baking powder into a mixing bowl. In a separate bowl, beat the eggs, coconut oil/butter and stevia together.
If the pear puree is cool, stir it into the eggs.
Gradually add the wet ingredients to the dry and stir until it forms a semi-runny batter.
Spoon into a muffin tray (it should make 6 muffins). Bake at 375 for 12-15 mins.

254. Xmas Chocolate Chip Cupcakes

Ingredients
1/2 c Coconut Flour
5 Eggs
2 Egg Whites
1/2 c Cashew Butter (or coconut oil for nut free)
1/2 t low sodium Salt
1/2 t Baking Soda
1/2 t Gluten Free Baking Powder
5 drops stevia liquid (May need a few more – please taste test)
3/4 c Egg Nog
1/4 t Vanilla
1/2 t Nutmeg
1 c Chocolate Chips
Vanilla Frosting
1 c coconut oil
2 T Canned Coconut Milk
1 t Vanilla

Instructions
Whisk together the dry ingredients.
Beat the eggs, whites, egg nog, butter, vanilla, and stevia. By 1/2 cup-fulls, add the dry mixture and whisk until smooth. Fold in the chocolate chips.
Preheat the oven to 350 degrees. Fill lined muffin tins 1/2 full with batter. Bake for 25-30 minutes, or until a toothpick.
If you want to do a loaf instead, bake in a loaf pan, same temp, for 50-55 mins.
For the frosting, beat all the ingredients till light and fluffy!

255. Boston Cream Pie Cupcake Bonanza

Vanilla Cream
Ingredients:
2 organic cage-free egg yolks
5 drops stevia liquid (May need a few more – please taste test)
2 tablespoons coconut palm sugar
2 tablespoons plus 1/2 teaspoon arrowroot starch/flour
pinch of pink low of sodium salt
1 cup canned coconut cream/milk, full fat, room temperature
1/2 teaspoon vanilla

Cupcakes
Ingredients:
1 & 1/2 cups fine blanched almond flour
1 & 1/2 teaspoons baking powder
1/2 teaspoon pink low sodium salt
1/2 cup canned coconut cream/milk, full fat, room temperature
6 tablespoons unsalted grass-fed butter, plus more for greasing
3 organic cage-free eggs
1 cup coconut palm sugar
1 teaspoon vanilla

Chocolate Ganache
Ingredients:
1 cup Enjoy Life Mini Chocolate Chips
1/4 cup canned coconut cream/milk, full fat, room temperature
4 tablespoons unsalted grass-fed butter
1 teaspoon vanilla

Directions:
1. Start by making the Vanilla Cream. In a small bowl whisk egg yolks together until smooth, set aside. In a medium saucepan combine stevia, coconut palm sugar, arrowroot, and salt and stir over medium heat. Add milk in a slow steady stream. Stir and let cook until the mixture begins to boil and thicken, about 5 minutes.
2. Pour 1/3 of the milk mixture into the yolks and stir together with a whisk until combined. Then pour back into the saucepan with the rest of the milk mixture and cook over medium heat, stirring often, until thick, about 3 minutes. Now stir in the vanilla.
3. Use a fine sieve to pour the vanilla mixture through into a small bowl. Cover it with plastic wrap and press the wrap down directly on to the surface of the cream. Refrigerate until very cold, an hour at least. While you wait prepare your cupcakes and chocolate ganache.
4. Preheat oven to 350. Grease a mini cupcake pan very liberally with butter. In a large bowl combine almond flour, baking powder and salt, use a fork to stir together. Warm coconut cream/milk and butter in a saucepan over low heat.
5. In a separate large bowl, whisk together eggs and coconut palm sugar. Then fold in the dry mixture.
6. Bring the coconut cream/milk and butter mixture to a boil. Add this mixture to the batter and whisk until smooth. Now stir in the vanilla. Pour batter into a Ziploc bag, cut a small hole in the corner. Transfer batter to prepared pan, filling to the top. Bake for 10-12 minutes or until a toothpick comes out clean. While you are waiting for the cupcakes to cool, go ahead and make your chocolate ganache.
7. Using the double boiler method melt together the chocolate, coconut cream/milk and butter. Once melted and combined stir in the vanilla. Transfer ganache to a Ziploc bag once it's cool enough, and cut a small hole in the corner tip.

8. Once your cupcakes are cool, remove two from the pan at a time. Squeeze a layer of vanilla cream over the top of one cupcake and then flip the other one upside down and use it to sandwich the two together. Then pour your chocolate ganache over the top and enjoy!

Notes:

You may have noticed above it says Coconut Cream or Coconut Milk. Coconut Cream can be found at health food stores like Sprouts or Whole Foods next to the regular coconut milk. I prefer it because it's a little thicker than normal coconut milk, so if you can find it use it, if not coconut milk will work just fine.

256. Vanilla Bean Cupcakes with Mocha Buttercream

Ingredients
 (makes 5-6 cupcakes):
For the cupcakes
1/4 cup coconut flour, sifted
1/4 teaspoon low sodium salt
1/8 teaspoon baking soda
Seeds scraped from half a vanilla bean
1/2 teaspoon vanilla extract
3 large eggs
1/4 cup coconut oil
5 drops stevia liquid (May need a few more – please taste test)

Insytructions
Preheat the oven to 350 and line a muffin tin with paper liners. Whisk together the coconut flour, salt, and baking soda in a medium bowl. Add the vanilla bean seeds, and mix together with your fingers, pinching the mixture to evenly distribute the vanilla seeds. In a small bowl, whisk together the vanilla extract, eggs, coconut oil, and stevia. Add the wet ingredients to the dry and whisk well, or beat with a hand mixer, until very smooth. Pour the batter into the cupcake cups and bake for 15-20 minutes, or until a toothpick comes out clean.
For the frosting:
8 tablespoons 1 stick) unsalted butter, at room temperature
5 drops stevia liquid (May need a few more – please taste test)
1 tablespoon cocoa
Tiny pinch of low sodium salt
1/4 teaspoon vanilla extract
1/4 teaspoon finely ground coffee
Coffee beans for garnish
Using a hand mixer, beat the butter until very smooth. Add the remaining ingredients and beat until incorporated. If your frosting does not seem stiff enough, refrigerate for a little while, then beat again. Once the cupcakes are completely cool, pipe or spread on the frosting (I used a Wilton 1M tip). Top with a coffee bean if desired.

257. Meaty Meatloaf Cupcakes

Ingredients
1.5-2 pounds of ground beef (grass-fed if possible)
3 eggs
¼ cup almond flour (or enough to thicken- this will depend partially on the fat content of the meat and the texture of the almond flour)
1 teaspoon dried basil
1 teaspoon garlic powder
1 medium onion
2 tablespoons worcestershire sauce
Salt and pepper to taste
5-6 sweet potatoes
¼ cup butter or coconut oil
1 teaspoon low sodium Salt

Instructions
Preheat the oven to 375 degrees
Finely dice the onion or puree in a blender or food processor.
In a large bowl, combine the meat, eggs, flour, basil, garlic powder, pureed onion, Worcestershire sauce, and salt and pepper and mix by hand until incorporated.
Grease a muffin tin with coconut oil or butter and evenly divide the mixture into the muffin tins to make 2-3 meat "muffins" per person. If you don't have a muffin tin, you can just press the mixture into the bottom of an 8x8 or 9x13 baking dish.
Put into oven on middle rack, and put a baking sheet with a rim under it, in case the oil from the meat happens to spill over (should only happen with fattier meats if at all)
For sweet potatoes: if they are small enough, you can put them into the oven at the same time, if not you can peel, cube and boil them until soft.
When meat is almost done, make sure sweet potatoes are cooked by whichever method you prefer, and drain the water if you boiled them.
Mix with butter and salt or pepper if desired and mash by hand or with an immersion blender.
Remove meat "muffins" from the oven when they are cooked through and remove from tin. Top each with a dollop of the mashed sweet potatoes to make it look like a cupcake.

Paleo Diet Recipes 365 Days of Paleo and Coconut Recipes by Mercedes Del Rey

258. Gushing Guava Cupcakes with Whipped Guava Frosting

Ingredients
For the Cake
¾ cup (120g) of Coconut Flour
¾ cup (96g) of Tapioca Flour
¾ cup of Light Olive Oil
6 Tablespoons (85g) of Granulated Sugar or Coconut Sugar
5 drops stevia liquid (May need a few more – please taste test)
½ cup of Concentrated Guava Puree ('applesauce thick')
6 Eggs
1 teaspoon of Lime Juice
1½ teaspoon of Cream of Tartar
¾ teaspoon of Baking Soda
½ teaspoon of low sodium Salt
For the Whipped Guava Frosting
¾ cup of room temperature coconut oil
6 Tablespoons of Concentrated Guava Puree ('applesauce thick')
5 drops stevia liquid (May need a few more – please taste test)
½ cup of Arrowroot Starch, sifted
1 teaspoon of Lime
Pinch of low sodium Salt

Instructions
For the Cake
You may have to boil the guava puree until applesauce thick. I used Goya brand and let it boil for about 10 minutes.
Preheat oven to 350F. We will drop the temperature to 325F to bake. Line the muffin tin with cupcake liners.
Separate the eggs into egg yolks and egg whites.
Combine the egg whites and cream of tartar and beat with a whisk attachment on high speed. Place the whites in a bowl and set aside, or store in the refrigerator while preparing the rest of the ingredients.
Combine the olive oil, egg yolks, stevia, lime juice, and guava puree in the mixing bowl and beat on high speed for about 30 seconds.
Sift together the coconut flour, tapioca flour, baking soda, sugar, and salt to make the dry flour mixture.
Add half of the dry flour mixture to the wet mixture and whip until the flours absorb and the batter becomes fluffy. Scrape the sides with a spatula to incorporate.
Add the rest of the dry flour mixture and beat on high speed with the whisk until combined and fluffy.
Scoop in a heaping of the egg white meringue and hand mix into the batter. Gently fold in the rest of the meringue until combined.
Portion the batter into each cake pan and place tin in the oven centered.
Reduce the temperature to 325F and for 25-30 minutes until an inserted toothpick comes out clean. This method will give a nice dome to the cupcakes and prevent over browning of the stevia.
Let cool to room temperature or colder before frosting.
For the Frosting
Chill the beaters and mixing bowl in the freezer for about 15 minutes.
Combine the raw stevia and guava puree in a cup until it forms a thicker syrup.
Whip the coconut shortening and optionally the cream cheese.

Add the arrowroot starch and salt and whip.
While mixing on medium speed, pour the guava mixture slowly. Whip until pink and pretty.
Add more stevia to taste if you like.
Dollop onto a cooled cupcake and enjoy!

259. Blushing Blueberry Muffin Recipe

Ingredients
2 1/2 cups almond flour
1 Tablespoon coconut flour
1/4 teaspoon low sodium salt
1/2 teaspoon baking soda
1 Tablespoon vanilla
1/4 cup coconut oil
5 drops stevia liquid (May need a few more – please taste test)
1/4 cup coconut milk*
2 eggs
1 cup fresh or frozen blueberries
2-3 Tablespoons cinnamon

Instructions
Preheat oven to 350. Line a 12 count muffin tin and lightly oil with coconut oil.
In a mixing bowl combine almond flour, coconut flour, salt, and baking soda and stir to combine.
Pour in coconut oil, eggs, stevia, coconut milk, and vanilla; mix well.
Fold in blueberries and add cinnamon.
Distribute into muffin tin. Sprinkle with additional cinnamon.
Bake for 22-25 minutes. Allow to cool and enjoy!

Notes
*Coconut milk can come in different textures depending on the brand you use. If you use a thicker brand like THAI, then use 1/8 cup of coconut milk and 4 Tablespoons of water. If your coconut milk is thinner, stick to the 1/4 cup of coconut milk.

260. Healthy Carrot Ginger Muffins

Ingredients:
2 cups blanched almond flour
½ teaspoon low sodium salt
1 teaspoon baking soda
½ tsp allspice
½ tsp powdered ginger
a pinch of clove
½ cup shredded coconut shreds, unsweetened
3 eggs, preferably pastured
½ cup coconut oil, melted
5 drops stevia liquid (May need a few more – please taste test)
1-2 Tbs grated fresh ginger
1 cup grated carrot
3/4 cup raisins, soaked in water for 15 minutes and drained

Instructions:
In a large bowl, combine almond flour, salt, baking soda, spices, and coconut shreds
In a smaller bowl whisk together eggs, oil, and syrup. Add fresh ginger, grated carrot, and raisins.
Stir wet ingredients into dry
Spoon batter into paper- lined muffin tins
Bake at 350° for 18-20 minutes for mini muffins OR 24-26 minutes for regular muffins.
Cool and serve.

261. Pecan Muffins

(makes 12)
Ingredients
1/3 cup coconut flour
1/4 cup butter, melted
3 large eggs
1/3 cup chopped pecans
1/4 tsp baking powder
stevia drops to taste
Instructions
Whisk together the butter, eggs and molasses.
Sieve the coconut flour and baking powder into a large mixing bowl.
Gradually add the wet ingredients to the dry, stirring until it forms a thick, runny Fold in the pecans.
Spoon about a tbsp into small (I used 4cm) muffin cups. It should stretch to 12. Bake at 350 for 10-12 minutes.

262. Temptingly Perfect Plantain Drop

Ingredients
3 tablespoons coconut oil
2 brown plantains (they must be brown)
1 tsp stevia
¼ cup coconut oil, melted
3 eggs
1 tablespoon canned coconut milk
3 tablespoons coconut flour
1-2 teaspoons cinnamon (I used 2 because I love cinnamon)
1 teaspoon baking powder
A pinch of low sodium salt

Instructions
1. Preheat oven to 350 degrees.
2. Cut the ends off of the plantains, then use your knife to cut them in half lengthwise and then peel the skin off, cutting off any excess skin that sticks to the plantains. The browner the plantains are, the sweeter they will be and the easier the skin is to take off.
3. Now place a large skillet over medium-high heat, add 3 tablespoons of coconut oil to heat up, then add the halved plantains to the skillet. Cook on both sides for about 3-4 minutes until browned, making sure not to burn them.
4. Once the plantains are done cooking, add them to the food processor and puree until they begin to clump together.
5. Then add the stevia, coconut oil, eggs, and coconut milk and puree until smooth. No clumps should be present at this point.
6. Now add coconut flour, cinnamon, baking powder, and salt to the food processor and puree one more time to combine everything well.
7. Now line a baking sheet with parchment paper and grab an ice cream scoop to help form perfect sized biscuits.
8. Scoop the batter out and plop each biscuit on the baking sheet about 1 inch away from each other. My batter made 8 biscuits.
9. Place in oven and bake for 20-25 minutes until slightly brown and completely cooked through.
10. Let cool. These babies are hot and need to settle afterwards.

263. Sweety Potato Muffins

Ingredients
1/2 c Coconut Flour
6 Eggs
2 t Vanilla
1 t low sodium Salt
1 t Baking Soda
2 t Cinnamon
1/2 c Ground Flax
2 Sweet Potatoes or Yams, baked and mashed (discard skins)
1 c Raisins or Chocolate Chips (optional)

Instructions:
Whisk together all the dry ingredients. Beat the eggs and add dry mix by spoonfuls until well blended. Add the mashed sweet potatoes.
Spoon batter into lined muffin cups. Bake at 350 degrees for 30-35 minutes.
Enjoy!

264. Zesty Zucchini Muffins

Ingredients
3/4 C applesauce
5 drops stevia liquid (May need a few more – please taste test)
1/4 C coconut oil, melted
3 eggs
1 Tbsp vanilla
2 C almond flour
1 1/2 tsp baking soda
1 C zucchini, shredded
3/4 C raisin

Instructions
With electric or stand mixer, beat applesauce, stevia and oil
Add eggs and vanilla and mix until combined
Slowly mix in almond flour and soda, then beat until batter forms
Fold in zucchini and raisins
Bake at 350 degrees for 25 minutes, makes 15 muffins

265. Cozy Coconut Flour Muffins

Ingredients
1/2 cup coconut flour
6 eggs, at room temperature (that's important)
¼ cup almond milk
2 tsp stevia
6 Tbs. coconut oil
2 Tbsp coconut milk at room temperature
2 tsp. vanilla extract
1/4 tsp. baking soda
1 tsp. apple cider vinegar

Instructions
Preheat the oven to 350 degrees and prepare a muffin tin with 8 liners (I like unbleached parchment paper baking cups).
Combine the coconut flour and eggs until smooth. Add the remaining ingredients and stir well.
Divide evenly between the muffin tins. Bake until golden and a toothpick comes out clean, about 20 minutes.
Cool completely.

**Makes 8 cupcakes. Feel free to double the recipe if you want more cupcakes! These last in an airtight container for a few days at room temperature. They also freeze really well!

Paleo Diet Recipes 365 Days of Paleo and Coconut Recipes by Mercedes Del Rey

266. Lemon Mousse Mouthwatering Cupcakes

Ingredients
1/2 cup coconut flour
6 eggs, at room temperature (that's important)
6 Tbs. milk
2 tsp stevia
6 Tbs. coconut oil
2 Tbs. coconut milk at room temperature
1 tsp. vanilla extract
1/2 tsp. ground cardamom
1/4 tsp. baking soda
1/2 tsp. apple cider vinegar
Instructions
Preheat the oven to 350 degrees and prepare a muffin tin with 8 liners (I like unbleached parchment paper baking cups).
Combine the coconut flour and eggs until smooth. Add the remaining ingredients and stir well.
Divide evenly between the muffin tins. Bake until golden and a toothpick comes out clean, about 20 minutes.
Cool completely and frost with the lemon mousse.
Makes 8 cupcakes. Feel free to double the recipe if you want more cupcakes!
Lemon Mousse Frosting
Ingredients
3/4 cup stevia-sweetened lemon curd (recipe below)
1 cup coconut milk
1 Tbs. light coconut milk
1 tsp stevia
Pinch of low sodium salt to taste
Instructions
First, make the stevia-sweetened lemon curd, by simply whisking the whole eggs, yolks and 1tsp stevia in a saucepan until smooth, then place pan over a low heat. Add the coconut oil, juice and zest and whisk continuously until thickened. Strain through a sieve. Lemon curd keeps, covered, in the fridge for 2 weeks. Chill until thickened and cold before using it.
In a small saucepan, whisk together the coconut milk and gelatin. Let it sit for 10 minutes. Then turn the heat on medium and whisk until the gelatin dissolves. Pour into a bowl and refrigerate until set, about 4 hours.
In a food processor, blend together the set coconut milk and the lemon curd until smooth. Add stevia to taste and a small pinch of low sodium salt.

267. Sexy Savory Muffins

Ingredients
½ cup coconut flour
1 tsp baking soda
½-1 tsp low sodium salt
¼ cup coconut oil
½ cup + 2 tbsp coconut milk
4 pastured eggs
1 tsp apple cider vinegar
1 tsp garlic powder
½ tsp each of rosemary, thyme, sage

Instructions
1. Pre-heat the oven to 350°. Melt the coconut oil and combine with remaining muffin ingredients in a food procssor or bowl, mix well.
2. Place batter in a muffine tin lined with muffin liners. The muffins will raise a small amount, so you can fill the muffin liner about ¾ full–almost to the top. Bake for about 20-30 minutes or until a toothpick inserted comes out clean and the tops are slightly browned.
3. Let it cool and slice in small squares.

268. Molten Lava Chocolate Cupcake

Ingredients:
4 oz Semi-Sweet or Bittersweet chocolate
½ tsp Vanilla Extract
1/8 tsp Salt
5 drops stevia liquid (May need a few more – please taste test)
1 tsp Coconut Flour
2 tsp Cacao Powder
2 eggs
4 Tbsp extra virgin coconut oil (plus a little more for greasing the ramekins)

Instructions:
1. Preheat oven to 375F. Grease four 6oz ramekins with coconut oil.
2. In a 4 cup measuring cup or medium microwave-safe bowl, melt chocolate and coconut oil in the microwave on low power. Stir until smooth and let cool.
3. In a small bowl, beat eggs, vanilla, salt and sugar with a hand mixer until light and frothy, about five minutes (this can seem like an eternity with a hand mixer, but hang in there because it's worth it!).
4. Pour egg mixture over chocolate. Sift cocoa and coconut flour over the top. Then gently fold all the ingredients together.
5. Pour batter into prepared ramekins (they should be filled to within ½" of the top). Place the ramekins on a baking sheet and place in the oven (you can chill the ramekins for a few hours if you want to make them ahead of time, just make sure you bring them back to room temperature before baking). Bake for 11-12 minutes.
6. Remove from oven and serve immediately. Enjoy!

269. Party Carrot Cupcakes

Ingredients
Wet
3 eggs
6 tablespoon non-dairy milk
6 tablespoon extra virgin coconut oil, melted
6 tablespoon carrot juice
5½ tablespoon egg whites
30 drops liquid stevia*see note
¾ teaspoon pure vanilla extract
Dry
6 tablespoon coconut flour
1 teaspoon baking powder
¼ teaspoon low sodium salt
pinch ground cinnamon

Instructions
Preheat oven to 350F and line 12 muffin tins with medium-sized paper liners.
Place eggs and egg white in blender and beat well, about 30 seconds. My magic bullet worked great for this!
Pour in carrot juice, milk, coconut oil, stevia and vanilla. Blend quickly to mix.
Drop in dry ingredients and mix for about 10 seconds. The batter should be slightly thicker than pancake batter.
Pour into prepared muffin tins and bake for 25-30 minutes or until inserted toothpick comes out clean. Mine took 26 minutes. Remove from pan and allow to cool on cooling rack for at least 1 hour before applying buttercream.

270. Cinnamon Chocolate Chip Muffins

Ingredients
Muffins
6 large eggs
5 drops stevia liquid (May need a few more – please taste test)
1 teaspoon vanilla extract
8 tablespoons (1 stick) unsalted butter, melted
3/4 cup coconut flour
1 tablespoon ground cinnamon
2 teaspoons baking powder
1 teaspoon baking soda
small pinch low sodium salt

Instructions
Muffins
Preheat oven to 375 fahrenheit and adjust rack to middle position
Line with muffin liners
Whisk eggs, stevia, vanilla, butter, and applesauce in a large mixing bowl or use a stand mixer
Sift coconut flour, cinnamon, baking powder, baking soda, and salt over a medium bowl
Add dry ingredients to wet ingredients and until well blended
Fold in chocolate chips ensuring an even distribution throughout your batter
Spoon batter into muffin cups and bake for 16-18 minutes, or until a toothpick in the center comes out clean
Remove the muffins from the oven and let cool
Once cool you can head below and make the frosting to go with them
Notes
*You can not let Coconut flour sit long, as soon as you mix this batter, ensure you put it right into the oven *If you want chocolate muffins, you can add between 1/4 - 1/2 cup of cocoa powder to your taste liking *You can store these in an airtight container for 3 days *You can substitute the butter with Coconut Oil but I haven't tested it and 8 tablespoons would probably be too oily. If you do test it, start with half and please let me know how it worked.

271. Strawberry Shortcake Cupcakes

Ingredients:
2½ cups blanched almond flour
¾ teaspoon baking soda
¼ teaspoon low sodium salt
5 drops stevia liquid (May need a few more – please taste test)
⅓ cup coconut oil, melted
4 large eggs, room temperature
1 tablespoon lemon juice
2 teaspoons vanilla extract
½ teaspoon lemon zest
½ cup finely chopped strawberries
Frosting
2 egg whites, room temperature
5 drops stevia liquid (May need a few more – please taste test)
¼ teaspoon lemon juice or vinegar
1½ tablespoons strawberry preserves (freshly pureed strawberries will work too)

Instructions:
Preheat the oven to 325 degrees F.
Line a standard muffin tin with baking cups.
Combine the stevia, coconut oil, eggs, lemon juice, vanilla, and lemon zest in the jar of a blender. Puree on medium speed for 20 seconds or until frothy and smooth.
Add the dry ingredients and blend on high for 30-45 seconds. The batter should be very smooth and contain no lumps. If needed, scrape down the sides with a spatula and blend again for a few seconds until all of the dry mixture is incorporated.
Gently fold the chopped strawberries in by hand. Divide the batter evenly into the muffin tin, filling about ¾ of the way full.
Bake for 16-18 minutes, until a toothpick can be inserted into the middle and comes out clean.
Let the cupcakes cool completely on the counter before frosting.
Frosting
Once the cupcakes have cooled, make your Italian meringue.
Bring your stevia to a boil in a saucepan over medium-high heat.
Meanwhile, beat the egg whites and lemon juice until frothy and you can just begin to see trail marks from your beaters. When you lift out the beaters, you should see soft peaks.
With the beaters or mixer running, slowly pour in the boiling stevia in a steady stream. Continue beating for 6-8 minutes, until the meringue is cool to the touch.
Gently fold in the strawberry preserves. Put the frosting into a piping bag for a pretty design, or spread onto cupcakes with a knife.
Tips
For easier separation, separate the whites from the yolks when they are cold.
Meringue will not stiffen if you use a dirty bowl (usually because of leftover oil) or let any of the yolk get in with the whites
Over beating will cause the meringue to fall. Stop once you can lift the beaters out and see stiff peaks.
The frosting needs to be piped immediately and is best served immediately as well. Once it's on the cupcakes though, it will hold up in the refrigerator for 24 hours.

272. Thin Mint Mini Cupcakes

Ingredients
For the Cupcakes
1/4 cup coconut flour
1/4 cup organic cocoa powder
4 large eggs (at room temperature)
1/4 cup coconut oil
5 drops stevia liquid (May need a few more – please taste test)
1/4 tsp baking soda
1 tsp lemon juice
Pinch of low sodium salt
1/4 tsp mint extract
6 Tbsp chopped dark chocolate or dairy free chocolate chips (for Paleo)

For the frosting:
2/3 cup powdered sweetener or coconut sugar, powdered for Paleo
2 ripe avocado
1/2 cup coconut milk
1/4 tsp mint extract

Instructions
Preheat oven to 350 F
Combine the coconut flour, cocoa powder, sweetener (if granular), baking soda, and low sodium salt.
In a separate bowl, combine the eggs, coconut oil, and lemon juice (and stevia if using).
Add the dry ingredients to the wet and mix to combine.
Line a mini muffin tin with 24 cupcake liners.
Fill cupcake liners evenly with the batter and bake for 13-15 minutes or until cooked through.
Allow to cool before topping with the icing.
Pipe on the frosting (directions below) onto each cupcake and serve.
For the frosting
Place the meat of the avocados in a blender and mix until completely smooth.
Add the sweetener, coconut milk, and mint extract. Mix until thoroughly incorporated.

Notes
Total Carb Count: 3.1 g (for 1 mini cupcake plus the carbs for the sweetener used)
Net Carb Count: 1.2 g net carbs (for 1 mini cupcake plus the carbs for the sweetener used)
*Note carb counts are estimated based on the products I used. Check nutrition labels for accurate carb counts and gluten information.

273. Lemon-Coconut Petit Fours

Ingredients
For the Cake
1/2 cup coconut flour
1/2 cup coconut milk
3 eggs, separated
3/4 cup soaked dates in 3 tbsp hot water
1/2 tsp vanilla
1/2 tsp baking soda
1/4 tsp low sodium salt
1 tsp lemon rind

Frosting
2/3 cup coconut cream (from the top of a can of coconut milk)
2 tbsp almond milk
1 tbsp Stevia
3 tsp lemon juice
¼ cup coconut oil, room temperature

Instructions
Put dates in a heat safe bowl or container and pour 3 tbsp boiling water over them and let soak for about 15 minutes. You can chop the dates before soaking to speed up the process, but it's not necessary.
Separate the eggs with yolks in one bowl and whites in one large stainless steel, glass or ceramic bowl. When you go to whip the egg whites, it helps if they are at room temperature.
Once dates have soaked put them in a food processor along with remaining water and mix until you have a paste-like consistency. Add coconut flour, milk, egg yolks, vanilla, baking soda, salt and lemon rind and mix.
Whip the egg whites until foamy and stiff peaks form. This is much easier if you have a stand mixer with the whisk attachment or a hand mixer. It is possible to do it by hand, but takes time.
Gently fold egg whites into the batter. Grease a standard sized loaf pan. Put batter in pan and even out the top with a spatula or spoon.
Bake in a 350° oven for 20-30 minutes or when a toothpick inserted comes out clean.

For the frosting
Coconut cream can be purchased in cans or you can skim the cream of the top of cans of coconut milk, however you may have to use multiple cans of coconut milk. Put coconut cream in a bowl and whisk for a few minutes to make it lighter and creamier.
Add coconut oil, milk, stevia and lemon juice and whisk until fully incorporated.
Allow the cake to cool completely before frosting. Once the cake has cooled, cut small squares or circles out of the cake and skim some cake off of the top with a knife to make it even. There will be leftover scraps, but they make a great snack! Cut the squares in half and frost the middle. You can use the prepared frosting, but it will be very thin.
Drizzle the prepared frosting over the small cake squares and use a spatula or knife to frost the sides evenly. Once you've frosted each petit fours, refrigerate to allow the frosting to harden. Top with a bit of lemon rind.

274. Blushing Blueberry Cupcakes

Ingredients:
1/2 cup almond flour
1/2 cup coconut flour
1/2 cup hazelnut flour
1 tbsp coconut sugar
1 tsp baking soda
¼ tsp low sodium salt
3 eggs
3 tbsp unsweetened almond milk
5 drops stevia liquid (May need a few more – please taste test)
1 tsp vanilla extract
½ cup blueberries
Instructions
Preheat oven to 350°.
Combine dry ingredients (both flours, sugar, baking soda, and salt) into a bowl and mix.
In a separate bowl, whisk eggs together; add milk, stevia and vanilla and stir.
Fold wet ingredients into dry ingredients.
Stir in the blueberries by hand.
Line muffin tin with muffin liners and spray each one with a bit of nonstick spray (optional but recommended).
Pour batter evenly to your cupcake tray
Bake for 10-15 minutes or until batter is no longer in liquid form.
Drizzle with extra stevia if desired.
Enjoy!

Paleo Diet Recipes 365 Days of Paleo and Coconut Recipes by Mercedes Del Rey

275. Delicious Morning Cupcakes

Ingredients
1/3 cup mashed sweet potato
3 eggs
¼ 5 drops stevia liquid (May need a few more – please taste test)
1 teaspoon pure vanilla extract
1 cup grated carrot (1 large)
1 cup grated apple (½ large Fugi)
2 teaspoons fresh ginger, peeled and grated, optional
2 cups blanched almond flour
1 cup unsweetened shredded coconut (or flaked coconut)
2/3 cup raisins
2/3 cup raw walnuts, chopped
2 teaspoons ground cinnamon
1 teaspoon baking powder
¼ teaspoon baking soda
½ teaspoon low sodium salt

Instructions
Preheat the oven to 350 degrees F and line a 12-cupcake tray with baking cups.
Whisk together the mashed sweet potato, eggs, stevia, grated carrot, apple, and ginger until well-combined (wet ingredients).
In a seperate mixing bowl, stir together the almond flour, raisins, walnuts, cinnamon, baking powder, baking soda, and salt (dry ingredients).
Pour the dry mixture into the bowl with the wet mixture and stir well until a thick batter forms.
using an ice cream scoop or small measuring cup, scoop batter into the lined muffin tray, filling the cups 3/4 of the way up.
Place cupcake tray on the center rack in the preheated oven and bake for 30 to 35 minutes, until cupcake test clean when poked with a toothpick.
Allow cupcakes to cool at least 20 minutes before mowing them down < - if you try to eat the cupcakes before letting them cool, they will stick to the cupcake cups like whoa.

276. Cheerful Coffee Cupcake

Cupcake Ingredients:
6 eggs
1/4 cup ghee
1/4 cup coconut flour
1/4 cup water chestnut flour 2 Tbsp grade B stevia 2 Tbsp vanilla
5 drops stevia liquid (May need a few more – please taste test)
1/4 tsp low sodium salt
1/2 tsp cinnamon

Topping Ingredients:
1/2 cup pecans (chopped)
5 drops stevia liquid (May need a few more – please taste test)
4 Tbsp ghee
2 Tbsp almond flour
1 tsp cinnamon
1/8 tsp low sodium salt

Instructions
Preheat oven to 350 degrees.
Put eggs in a large mixing bowl and mix thoroughly with an immersion blender until frothy.
Add remaining ingredients and mix well.
Fill muffin pan evenly (should make 1 dozen).
Place in oven and set timer for 20 minutes.
Now combine ingredients for the topping in a separate bowl.
At the 20 minute mark take out the muffins and add the topping evenly between all the muffins.
Put them back in the oven for another 10 minutes.
Broil for an additional 2 minutes and remove quickly.
Let cool.
Enjoy with a hot cup of coffee! Ok, I guess I'll let you do tea if you insist

277. Luscious Lemon Poppy Seed Cupcake

Ingredients
1 1/4 cup almond flour
2 tbs coconut flour
1 tbs poppy seeds
1 tsp baking soda
1 tsp baking powder
1/4 tsp low sodium salt
5 drops stevia liquid (May need a few more – please taste test)
1/4 cup fresh lemon juice, plus the zest of 1 lemon
3 eggs whisked
3 tbs coconut oil
1 tsp vanilla extract

Instructions
Preheat oven to 350-degrees F
In a small bowl, mix all the wet ingredients together
In a medium bowl, combine all the dry ingredients
Now pour the wet ingredients into the dry ingredients bowl, and stir into a batter
Let batter set for a few minutes, then stir it again
Grease a muffin tin or use muffin liners and fill each well or cup about two-thirds full
Bake about 15-20 minutes, or until a toothpick inserted into a muffin comes out clean
Serve and enjoy!

278. Strawberry chia Cupcake

Ingredients
½ c + 2 tbsp (56g) coconut flour
1 tsp xanthan gum
¾ tsp baking powder
¾ tsp baking soda
¼ tsp low sodium salt
1 tbsp (13g) chia seeds
1 tbsp (5g) lemon zest (about one medium)
1 tbsp (14g) coconut oil or unsalted butter, melted
1 large egg, room temperature
1 tsp vanilla extract
¼ c (60g) plain nonfat Greek yogurt
¼ c (60mL) agave
3 tbsp (45mL) freshly squeezed lemon juice (about one medium-large)
½ c (120mL) unsweetened vanilla almond milk
2 scoops (84g) vanilla protein powder
1 c (140g) frozen unsweetened strawberries, thawed slightly and diced

Instructions
Preheat the oven to 350°F, and lightly coat 9 standard-sized muffin cups with nonstick cooking spray.
Whisk together the coconut flour, xanthan gum, baking powder, baking soda, salt, chia seeds, and lemon zest in a medium bowl. In a separate bowl, whisk together the coconut oil or butter, egg, and vanilla. Stir in the Greek yogurt until no large lumps remain. Stir in the agave, lemon juice, and almond milk. Mix in the protein powder. Add in the coconut flour mixture, stirring until fully incorporated. Let the batter rest for 10 minutes. Gently fold in the diced strawberries
Divide the batter between the prepared muffin cups. Bake at 350°F for 25-28 minutes, or until a toothpick inserted into the center comes out clean. Cool in the pan for 10 minutes before carefully turning out onto a wire rack.

Notes: Any milk (cow, soy, cashew, etc.) may be used in place of the almond milk.

279. Triple Coconut Cupcakes

Ingredients
1 cup almond flour
3 tbsp coconut flour
1 cup shredded coconut
1½ tsp baking powder
¼ tsp low sodium salt
5 drops stevia liquid (May need a few more – please taste test)
4 eggs, separated
¼ cup coconut oil
1 tbsp vanilla extract

Instructions
Preheat the oven to 350F. Grease a muffin tin or line with muffin cups.
Combine almond flour, coconut flour, shredded coconut, salt and baking powder in a medium mixing bowl.
Mix the egg yolks, stevia, coconut oil and vanilla extract in a small mixing bowl. Add to the almond flour mixture and combine thoroughly.
Using a hand mixer, whip the egg whites until they form stiff peaks.
Stir the egg whites into the rest of the ingredients, spoon the batter into the muffin tin.
Bake for 25 minutes (or until the tops are nicely browned and a tester comes out clean.

280. Lemon-Coconut Muffins

Ingredients
1 1/4 cup almond flour
1 cup shredded unsweetened coconut
2 tbs coconut flour
1/2 tsp baking soda
1/2 tsp baking powder
1/4 tsp low sodium salt
5 drops stevia liquid (May need a few more – please taste test)
1/3 cup fresh lemon juice, plus the zest of 1 lemon
1/4 cup full-fat coconut milk
3 eggs, whisked
3 tbs coconut oil
1 tsp vanilla extract

Instructions
Preheat oven to 350º F
In a small bowl, mix all the wet ingredients together
In a medium bowl, combine all the dry ingredients
Now pour the wet ingredients into the dry ingredients bowl, and stir into a batter
Let batter set for a few minutes, then stir it again
Grease a muffin tin or use silicone muffin liners (paper liners not recommended) and fill each well or cup about two-thirds full
Bake about 18-23 minutes. Test for doneness > insert toothpick into muffin center; if it comes out clean they're done
Serve and enjoy!

Paleo Diet Recipes 365 Days of Paleo and Coconut Recipes by Mercedes Del Rey

281. Chocolate Banana Muffins

Ingredients
2 medium super ripe bananas (each banana was 185 grams with the peel and 143 grams without)
5 drops stevia liquid (May need a few more – please taste test)
2 teaspoon vanilla extract
2 eggs
1/4 cup (56 grams) refined coconut oil, melted
200 grams (~2 cups but please weigh!) blanched almond flour
3 tablespoons (27 grams) coconut flour
1/3 cup (42 grams) Dutch process cocoa powder
1 teaspoon baking soda
1/4 teaspoon low sodium salt
1 cup (180 grams) semi-sweet chocolate chips ,additional mini chocolate chips for sprinkling, if desired

Directions
Preheat the oven to 350°F (175°C) and line a muffin tin with 12 muffin liners.
In a large bowl, mash the bananas with the bottom of a glass. They should almost be like a puree.
Add the stevia and vanilla and stir.
Add in the eggs and oil and stir until well combined.
In a medium bowl, mix together the almond flour, coconut flour, cocoa powder, baking soda and salt.
Stir just until combined and then stir in the chocolate chips.
Spoon the batter into the muffin liners and sprinkle on additional chocolate chips, if desired.
Bake for 18 minutes or until a toothpick inserted in the center comes out clean. Be careful not to confuse a melted chocolate chip with the batter.
Let the muffins cool for 5 minutes in the pan and then turn out onto a wire rack to cool completely.
Place in an airtight container and store in the refrigerator for up to 5 days.
Notes
Use can use unrefined coconut oil if you don't mind a slight coconut taste.

282. Delicious English Cupcakes

Ingredients
For the regular option
¼ cup almond or cashew flour
1 tablespoon coconut flour
¼ teaspoon baking soda
⅛ teaspoon low sodium salt
1 egg
½ tablespoon coconut oil
2 tablespoons water
For the cinnamon raisin option add the following to the regular option above
¼ teaspoon cinnamon
½ 5 drops stevia liquid (May need a few more – please taste test)
1½ tablespoons golden raisins
Instructions
Whisk together the dry ingredients in a small bowl.
Add the remaining wet ingredients and whisk again until fully incorporated.
Transfer the mixture into a greased microwave safe ramekin
Microwave for 2 minutes.
Remove from the ramekin, slice the muffin in half and toast for 2-3 minutes in a toaster oven.
Serve with softened butter.

283. Amazing Almond Flour Cupcakes

Ingredients:
2-1/2 cups almond flour or almond meal
¾ tsp baking soda
½ tsp low sodium salt
3 large eggs
⅓ cup unsweetened pumpkin puree, thawed winter squash puree, butternut squash puree, unsweetened apple sauce, or mashed very ripe banana
2 drops stevia, agave nectar or stevia
2 tablespoons coconut oil (melted) or vegetable oil
1 teaspoon vinegar (white or cider)
Optional Flavorings: 1 teaspoon extract (e.g., vanilla, almond), citrus zest, dried herbs (e.g., basil, dill), or spice (e.g., cinnamon, cumin)
Optional Stir-Ins: 1 cup fresh fruit (e.g., blueberries, diced apple) or ½ cup dried fruit/cacao nibs/chopped nuts/seeds or
Instructions:
Preheat oven to 350F. Line 10 cups in a standard 12-cup muffin tin with paper or foil liners.
In a large bowl whisk the almond flour, baking soda and salt (whisk in any dried spices or herbs at this point, if using).
In a small bowl, whisk the eggs, pumpkin, stevia, oil and vinegar (add any extracts or zest at this point, if using).
Add the wet ingredients to the dry ingredients, stirring until blended. Fold in any optional stir-ins, if using.
Divide batter evenly among prepared cups.
Bake in preheated oven for 14 to 18 minutes until set at the centers and golden brown at the edges. Move the tin to a cooling rack and let muffins cool in the tin 30 minutes. Remove muffins from tin.

284. Delightful Cinnamon Apple Muffins

Ingredients:
1 cup unsweetened applesauce
4 eggs
1/4 cup coconut oil, melted
1 tsp vanilla
Stevia to taste
1/2 cup coconut flour
2 tsp cinnamon
1 tsp baking powder
1 tsp baking soda
1/4 tsp low sodium salt

Instructions:

Preheat oven to 350 degrees F. Line a muffin tin with liners. In a large bowl, add applesauce, eggs, coconut oil, stevia, and vanilla. Stir to combine.

Stir in the coconut flour, cinnamon, baking powder, baking soda, and low sodium salt. Distribute the batter evenly into the lined muffin tins, filling each about two-thirds of the way full.

Bake for 15-20 minutes, until a toothpick inserted into the center comes out clean. Serve warm or store in the refrigerator in a resealable bag.

285. Delish Banana Nut Muffins

Ingredients:
4 bananas, mashed with a fork (the more ripe, the better)
4 eggs
1/2 cup almond butter
2 tbsp coconut oil, melted
1 tsp vanilla
1/2 cup coconut flour
2 tsp cinnamon
1/2 tsp nutmeg
1 tsp baking powder
1 tsp baking soda
1/4 tsp low sodium salt

Instructions:
Preheat oven to 350 degrees F. Line a muffin tin with cups. In a large bowl, add bananas, eggs, almond butter, coconut oil, and vanilla. Using a hand blender, blend to combine.

Add in the coconut flour, cinnamon, nutmeg, baking powder, baking soda, and low sodium salt. Blend into the wet mixture, scraping down the sides with a spatula. Distribute the batter evenly into the lined muffin tins, filling each about two-thirds of the way full.

Bake for 20-25 minutes, until a toothpick comes out clean. Serve warm or store in the refrigerator in a resealable bag.

286. Apple Cinnamon Muffins

Ingredients
5 eggs
1 cup homemade applesauce (store bought should work too)
½ cup coconut flour
2-3 TBSP cinnamon
1 tsp baking soda
1 tsp vanilla (optional)
¼ cup coconut oil
5 drops stevia liquid (May need a few more – please taste test)

Instructions
Preheat the oven to 400 degrees F.
Grease a muffin pan with coconut oil.
Put all ingredients into a medium sized bowl and mix with immersion blender or whisk until well mixed.
Let sit 5 minutes.
Use ⅓ cup measure to spoon into muffin tins.
Bake 12-15 minutes until starting to brown and not soft when lightly touched on the top.
Let cool 2 minutes, drizzle with honey (if desired) and serve.

287. Apple Cardamom Cupcakes

Ingredients
½ cup applesauce
⅓ cup honey
4 large eggs
¼ cup coconut flour
½ teaspoon baking soda
¼ teaspoon salt
1 teaspoon cinnamon
¼ teaspoon nutmeg
¼ teaspoon cloves
½ teaspoon cardamom
For frosting:
1 cup coconut milk
1 cup honey
pinch of salt
1 teaspoon vanilla
2 tablespoons arrowroot powder
1 tablespoon water
1 cup coconut oil, melted

Instructions
Preheat oven to 350 degrees. Prepare muffin/cupcake pan with liners.
Using an electric mixer or by hand, combine applesauce, honey, and eggs until smooth.
Sift together all dry ingredients, making sure to get out any lumps in the coconut flour.
Combine dry and wet ingredients, mixing thoroughly.
Divide batter amongst 10-12 cupcake liners, filling each one about ⅔ of the way up.
Place in oven and bake for 35-45 minutes, or until top is lightly browned and toothpick comes out clean.
Meanwhile, begin making frosting. In a medium saucepan, heat coconut milk, honey, salt, and vanilla and allow to simmer for 10 minutes.
In a small bowl or ramekin, combine arrowroot powder and water to form a thick paste.
Add arrowroot mixture to pan, whisk vigorously, and bring to a boil.
Remove pan from heat and very slowly add melted coconut oil while mixing with an electric hand blender.
Allow pan to cool slightly, then place whole thing in refrigerator for at least an hour or until it is cool and has turned white.
Remove from refrigerator and use electric hand blender to whip until fluffy.
Spread a dollop on each cupcakes (this frosting is quite sweet, so you don't need a lot but let your tastes be the guide!).
Sprinkle with cinnamon for garnish.

288. Chocolate Olive Oil Cupcakes

Ingredients
2 tablespoons cocoa powder
2 tablespoons coconut flour
1 teaspoon baking powder
1/4 teaspoon ground cinnamon
2 eggs
3 tablespoons honey
1/2 teaspoon vanilla extract
2 tablespoons olive oil
Icing
1 tablespoon coconut oil (melted)
1 tablespoon cocoa powder
1 tablespoon honey
Instructions for Cake
Preheat oven to 160 C.
Combine the cocoa, coconut flour, baking powder and cinnamon.
Add the eggs, honey, vanilla and olive oil.
Mix until smooth and well combined.
Spoon 4 lined cup cake tins.
Bake cupcakes for about 20 – 25 minutes.
Remove from the oven and allow to cool.
Instructions for Icing
Melt the coconut oil.
Mix in the cocoa powder.
Mix in the honey until all well combined.
Allow to harder then spread over muffins.
(Note: I didn't wait long enough for the icing to harder and the cupcake drank it up but it still tasted great!)

758   Pretty Vanilla Cup Cake
Ingredients
For the cupcakes:
¾ cup coconut flour
6 large eggs
¾ cup raw honey
½ cup melted coconut oil
1 tablespoon pure vanilla extract
¾ tsp baking powder
¼ tsp salt
For the icing:
1 can coconut milk (full fat) refrigerated overnight, scoop out coconut cream
1 tsp pure vanilla extract
2 heaping tablespoons pure coconut palm sugar or cane sugar
Instructions
Preheat the oven to 350 degrees.
Using a muffin pan, line each cup with a cupcake liner and spray generously with olive oil cooking spray or if not using cupcake liners grease very well with melted coconut oil.

In a bowl add the dry cupcake ingredients and mix to combine. In another small bowl whisk together the wet cupcake ingredients and add to the dry. Mix until completely smooth.

Pour the batter equally among the greased cups and bake in the oven for 16-18 minutes.

Allow the cupcakes to cook completely before removing from tin or removing from liners.

While the cupcakes are baking add the coconut cream to a large bowl with the vanilla and sugar. Use an electric beater and whip until frothy. Place in the fridge to chill.

Wait until the cupcakes are completely cooled and then pipe the coconut cream on each cupcake.

Place cupcakes back in the fridge for 3-4 hours to chill and the icing will firm up.

Top each cupcake with a halved fig slice, sprinkles, or other garnish of choice.

289. One-Bowl Coconut Flour Cupcakes

Ingredients
½ cup coconut flour
½ teaspoon baking powder
¼ teaspoon fine sea salt
4 large eggs (preferably brought to room temperature)
½ cup maple syrup, honey or agave nectar
⅓ cup coconut oil, warmed until melted (or vegetable oil of choice)
2 tablespoons dairy or nondairy milk of choice milk
2 teaspoons vanilla extract vanilla extract

Instructions
Preheat oven to 350°F.
IMPORTANT: Line 8 muffin cups with paper or silicone liners; spray insides of cups with nonstick cooking spray or oil/grease (to prevent sticking).
In a large bowl, whisk the flour, baking powder, and salt until blended. Whisk in the eggs, syrup, oil, milk, and vanilla until completely blended and smooth.
Divide the batter equally among the prepared muffin cups.
Bake in preheated oven for 18 to 22 minutes or until golden and a toothpick inserted in the center comes out clean.
Transfer baking tin to wire rack and cool 10 minutes.
Carefully remove the cupcakes from the tin and place on wire rack; cool completely.

Notes
Sore in an airtight container at room temperature for up to 2 days, in an airtight container in the refrigerator for up to 1 week, or freeze (unfrosted) for up to 2 months.

290. Meatloaf Cupcakes

Ingredients
1.5-2 pounds of ground beef (grass-fed if possible)
3 eggs
¼ cup almond flour (or enough to thicken- this will depend partially on the fat content of the meat and the texture of the almond flour)
1 teaspoon dried basil
1 teaspoon garlic powder
1 medium onion
2 tablespoons Worcestershire sauce
Salt and pepper to taste
5-6 sweet potatoes
¼ cup butter or coconut oil
1 teaspoon sea salt or Himalayan Salt

Instructions
Preheat the oven to 375 degrees
Finely dice the onion or puree in a blender or food processor.
In a large bowl, combine the meat, eggs, flour, basil, garlic powder, pureed onion, Worcestershire sauce, and salt and pepper and mix by hand until incorporated.
Grease a muffin tin with coconut oil or butter and evenly divide the mixture into the muffin tins to make 2-3 meat "muffins" per person. If you don't have a muffin tin, you can just press the mixture into the bottom of an 8x8 or 9x13 baking dish.
Put into oven on middle rack, and put a baking sheet with a rim under it, in case the oil from the meat happens to spill over (should only happen with fattier meats if at all)
For sweet potatoes: if they are small enough, you can put them into the oven at the same time, if not you can peel, cube and boil them until soft.
When meat is almost done, make sure sweet potatoes are cooked by whichever method you prefer, and drain the water if you boiled them.
Mix with butter and salt or pepper if desired and mash by hand or with an immersion blender.
Remove meat "muffins" from the oven when they are cooked through and remove from tin. Top each with a dollop of the mashed sweet potatoes to make it look like a cupcake.

291. Gluten Free Banana Nut Bread

Ingredients:
3 bananas, mashed, or 1 cup
3 eggs
1/2 cup almond butter
1/4 cup coconut oil, melted
1 tsp vanilla extract
1/2 cup almond flour
1/2 cup coconut flour
2 tsp cinnamon
1 tsp baking soda
1/4 tsp low sodium salt
1/2 cup chopped walnuts

Instructions:
Preheat the oven to 350 degrees F. Line a loaf pan with parchment paper. In a large bowl, add the mashed bananas, eggs, almond butter, coconut oil, and vanilla. Use a hand blender to combine.

In a separate bowl, mix together the almond flour, coconut flour, cinnamon, baking soda, and low sodium salt. Blend the dry ingredients into the wet mixture, scraping down the sides with a spatula. Fold in the walnuts.

Pour the batter into the loaf pan in an even layer. Bake for 50-60 minutes, until a toothpick inserted into the center comes out clean. Place the bread on a cooling rack and allow to cool before slicing.

292. Pumpkin crepes

ingredients
Apple Butter:
apples - 5 lb, peeled and sliced
cinnamon - to taste
Crepes:
egg yolk - 1
egg whites - 4
pure pumpkin puree - 1/3 cup
canned full-fat coconut milk - 1/3 cup
coconut flour - 3-4 tablespoons
arrowroot starch - 1/4 cup
pure vanilla extract - 1 teaspoon
ground allspice - 1/4 teaspoon
pure maple syrup - 3 tablespoons
instructions
Preheat oven to 425 degrees Fahrenheit.
Combine the apples and cinnamon to taste on 2 9 inch by 13 inch baking dishes.
Roast for 1-2 hours, stirring every 15 minutes, or until the apples have lost quite a bit of moisture.
Puree until smooth, adding water if necessary.
Preheat a nonstick skillet to 350 degrees Fahrenheit. Whisk together all crepe ingredients in a large bowl until smooth.
Lightly grease the skillet with coconut oil and add 4-5 tablespoons of batter, spreading it around with the back of a spoon.
Cook until the batter looks dry. Flip and cook until golden. Repeat with remaining batter.
Serve crepes with apple butter.

293. Red Coconut Smoothie

INGREDIENTS
1 cup coconut milk
1 frozen banana, sliced
2 cups frozen strawberries
1 teaspoon vanilla extract

INSTRUCTIONS
Add all ingredients to Blendtec and blend until smooth.

Paleo Diet Recipes 365 Days of Paleo and Coconut Recipes by Mercedes Del Rey

294. Briana's House Low Carb Chocolate Chip Cookies

INGREDIENTS
½ cup Briana's Baking Mix
½ cup oat fiber (use gluten free if necessary)
1 T THM Super Sweet Blend (or more to taste)
1 tsp. xanthan gum
½ tsp. baking soda
½ tsp. salt
8 T salted butter
4 T refined coconut oil
2 oz. cream cheese (full fat or reduced fat)
2 eggs
1 tsp. molasses
½ tsp. vanilla extract
¼ cup water
2 T heavy whipping cream
½ cup sugar free chocolate chips (such as Lily's brand) or chopped 85% dark chocolate

INSTRUCTIONS
Whisk the dry ingredients together.
Soften the butter, coconut oil, and cream cheese together, then beat them with the eggs, molasses, and vanilla until smooth. Add the water and whipping cream and beat again.
Add the dry ingredients to the wet ingredients and mix well. Stir in the chocolate chips by hand. Drop the dough by rounded tablespoons onto a cookie sheet, then smooth each cookie out thinly with the back of a spoon (each will be about 4 inches in diameter). Bake each pan of cookies at 375 degrees F for 7 minutes, then remove the pan from the oven and leave the cookies on it for 2 more minutes before transferring them to wire racks to cool completely. Store in the refrigerator. Yields 2 dozen cookies.
NOTES
Do not put cookie batter onto hot cookie sheets as you won't be able to spread the cookies out as well. Adjust the baking time according to how you like your cookies. This time is what worked best for me.

295. Coconut Vanilla Surprise

INGREDIENTS
1½ cups unflavored soy milk
2 tbsp. matcha green tea powder
stevia to taste
½ tsp. vanilla extract
¼ cup coconut milk
few dashes nutmeg

INSTRUCTIONS
Whisk together soy milk, matcha, sweetener and vanilla. Heat to desired temperate in a small saucepan on stove top or microwave in a microwave safe container.
Divide into mugs and froth.
Add coconut milk, and sprinkle with nutmeg. Serve.

296. Tempting Coconut Berry Smoothie

Ingredients:
½ Cup Frozen Blackberries
½ Frozen Banana
1 Teaspoon Chia Seeds
¼ Inch Piece Of Fresh Ginger
½ Cup Almond
Coconut Milk
1 scoop of HEMP protein
2 Tablespoons Toasted Coconut
Instructions:
Combine all the ingredients in a blender and process until smooth.

297. Pineapple Coconut Deluxe Smoothie

Ingredients:
1 C pineapple chunks
1 C coconut milk
1/2 C pineapple juice
1 ripe banana
1/2 – 3/4 C ice cubes
Pure liquid stevia to taste
1 tablespoon hemp protein powder

Instructions:
In a blender, combine the pineapple chunks, coconut milk, banana, ice and pure liquid stevia.
Puree until smooth.
Pour into 2 large glasses.
Garnish with a pineapple wedge if desired.

298. Sumptuous Strawberry Coconut Smoothie

Ingredients:
1 cup coconut milk
1 frozen banana, sliced
2 cups frozen strawberries
1 teaspoon vanilla extract
1 tablespoon hemp protein powder

Instructions:
Add all ingredients to blender and blend until smooth.

299. Divine Peach Coconut Smoothie

Ingredients:
1 cup full fat coconut milk, chilled
1 cup ice
2 large fresh peaches, peeled and cut into chunks
Fresh lemon zest, to taste
1 tablespoon hemp protein powder

Instructions:
Add coconut milk, ice and peaches blender. Using a zester, add a few gratings of fresh lemon zest. Blend on high speed until smooth.

300. Raspberry Coconut Smoothie

Ingredients:
½ - 1 cup coconut milk (depending on how thick you like it)
1 medium banana, peeled sliced and frozen
2 teaspoons coconut extract (optional)
1 cup frozen raspberries
1 tablespoon hemp protein powder

optional: shredded coconut flakes, and stevia to taste

Instructions:
Add coconut milk, frozen banana slices and coconut extract to your blender.
Pulse 1-2 minutes until smooth.
Add frozen raspberries and continue to pulse until smooth.
Pour into your serving glass, top with a couple of raspberries and a little shredded coconut, and enjoy!

301. Sweet Melon

Ingredients
1/2 honeydew melon, cut into chunks (about 4 cups, or 1 1/2 lbs)
1/2 cup light coconut milk
1-2 leaves fresh mint (plus more for garnish)
1/2-1 tsp. fresh lime juice (or to taste)
1 cup ice
Drizzle of honey or coconut nectar, to taste (optional, depending on how sweet your melon is)

Directions
Cut your melon in half, remove the seeds, and slice away the outer rind. Cut the melon into chunks, and add to your blender along with the coconut milk, mint, lime, and ice. Blend until smooth. Taste, and adjust sweetness with honey or coconut nectar. Serve with a garnish of mint, or fresh melon slices.

302. CINNAMON Coconut Surprise

Ingredients
1/2 Cup Coconut Milk
4 Large Egg Yolks
1 Medium Banana
1/4 Cup Ice
1/2 tsp Cinnamon
Directions
Throw all of the ingredients into your high-speed blender and blast for 30 to 60 seconds until well combined. Enjoy right away while still fresh, and give a little stir if separation occurs.

303. Low Carb Fried Zucchini

INGREDIENTS:
3 medium zucchini or yellow squash
2 eggs
1 tablespoon water
1/3 cup coconut flour
1/4 cup powdered Parmesan cheese
vegetable oil, for frying
ranch dressing, for serving

DIRECTIONS:
Heat a 1/4 inch of oil in the bottom of a large skillet over medium heat.
Wash and slice the zucchini into thin rounds, about 1/8-1/4 inch thick.
Beat together the egg and water in a shallow bowl.
Stir together the coconut flour and Parmesan in a second shallow bowl.
Coat the zucchini in the egg and then dredge in the coconut mixture to coat.
Add a single layer of zucchini to the hot oil, being careful not to crowd the pan. Fry for 1-2 minutes on each side, until golden brown. Repeat with remaining zucchini.
Drain on a paper towel lined plate. Sprinkle with salt, if desired.
Serve with ranch dressing for dipping.

Paleo Diet Recipes 365 Days of Paleo and Coconut Recipes by Mercedes Del Rey

304. Slow Cooker Paleo Mexican Breakfast Casserole

Ingredients
1 sweet potato, cubed or shredded
8 eggs, whisked
1/2 pound turkey bacon
1 yellow onion, chopped
1 red bell pepper, chopped
1 (8 ounce) package mushrooms, chopped (optional)
1/2 packet taco seasoning (or make your own if you're strict paleo!)
Guacamole, salsa and jalapeno to garnish

Instructions
Fry turkey bacon in a skillet until crispy. Remove and set aside. Crumble when cool enough to touch.
In the same skillet, cook the onions until they are soft.
Transfer the bacon, onions, sweet potato, bell pepper, mushrooms and eggs to the slow cooker. Stir to combine.
Sprinkle in your taco seasoning and stir again to dissolve.
Cook on LOW for 6-8 hours. Slice and serve with guacamole, salsa and jalapeno!

305. Paleo Pumpkin Pie Smoothie

Ingredients
1 frozen banana
2 tbsp pumpkin puree
½ cup unsweetened almond milk
½ tsp vanilla extract
1 tsp honey
1 tbsp hemp hearts
¼ tsp cinnamon
¼ tsp cloves
¼ tsp nutmeg

Instructions
Combine all ingredients in a blender and process until smooth. I find it's easier on the blender if I break the frozen banana into smaller chunks before processing.
Pour into a tall glass and enjoy with your favourite book, your favourite music, or both!

Notes
Calories: 220
Total Fat: 6.4g
Saturated Fat: 0.8g
Carbs: 38.0g
Fiber: 6.1g
Protein: 5.6g

306. Paleo Cookie Butter

Ingredients
For the Cookie Butter
½ cup (128 grams) favorite nut butter, almond, cashew or macadamia
½ cup (128 grams) roasted sunflower butter, such as SunButter®
½ cup (128 grams) raw organic coconut butter, such as Artisana®
¼ cup (60 grams) organic ghee (you could also use coconut oil)
4 tablespoons (84 grams) organic raw honey*
1½ tablespoons (20 grams) 100% pure cocoa butter, I use Callebaut®, melted
1½ tablespoons (10.5 grams) organic coconut flour, such as Tropical Traditions®
1 teaspoon (5 grams) unsulphured molasses, such as Brer Rabbit®
1 teaspoon (about 2 grams) pure vanilla extract, such as Nielsen-Massey®
½ to 1 teaspoon ground cinnamon, such as Penzey's® Cinnamon
¼ teaspoon ground allspice
¼ teaspoon freshly grated whole nutmeg
Generous pinch of fine sea salt
Coconut palm sugar or pure stevia extract powder, to taste

*Do not serve raw honey to children under the age of 1 year.

For the Optional Mix-Ins for "Cookie Dough Butter"
Chopped dark chocolate 70% cocoa or more
Gluten free semi-sweet chocolate chips, such as Trader Joe's®
Chopped walnuts or pecans, toasted or not
Unsweetened shredded coconut, toasted or not

Special Equipment
Mini Prep Food Processor
Mason jar with lid, helpful but not necessary
Rubber spatula
Preparation
Place nut butter and SunButter into work bowl of prep food processor.
In a small saucepan over medium-low heat, melt and brown the coconut butter and ghee until golden brown, stirring constantly, about 3 minutes for a lighter "blonde" browned coconut butter or 5 minutes for a darker, rich browned coconut butter the color of dark coffee and cream. (The mixture will bubble and foam. Keep stirring.) Remove immediately from heat to prevent overbrowning or burning; stir and allow to cool until still warm (not room temp, but no longer hot). Note: It is important to remove the pan immediately when coconut butter mixture is browned to desired doneness as the residual heat will continue to cook the mixture.
Add browned coconut butter mixture to nut butter and SunButter®; process until well combined and smooth scraping down sides of bowl as necessary between pulses. The mixture will be very thin at this point. Do not worry. Add honey, melted cocoa butter, coconut flour, molasses, vanilla extract, spices and salt; process until well combined and smooth. Taste and, if desired, sweeten additionally with coconut palm sugar or pure stevia extract.
Remove work bowl from processor unit. With a rubber spatula, or the plastic spatula that came with your processor unit, scrape and pour mixture into a small to medium bowl. Cover bowl with plastic food wrap and place in refrigerator until thickened, about 1 hour. Stir halfway through chilling time for an even chill. Remove from the fridge and stir to loosen.

Transfer to Mason® jar, if desired, or other covered container for storing. Before serving add and stir in favorite mix-ins as desired, about a few tablespoons each. Keep stored in an airtight container, such as a Mason® jar, in refrigerator.

Notes

Tip: This homemade cookie butter softens upon room temperature. If you wish for a thicker cookie butter, either keep it chilled or simply stir in an additional 1 tablespoon of coconut flour (or more to desired thickness).

307. Paleo-friendly Coconut Chocolate Coffee Cake

Ingredients
What you'll need:
(all ingredients are available at Whole Foods or Natural Grocers/health sections; my ordering recommendations listed)
two medium-sized glass bowls for mixing & one square glass baking dish (8"x8")
coconut oil for greasing baking dish
4 eggs
½ cup full-fat coconut milk
¼ cup coconut butter
½ cup brewed coffee or espresso, as strong as you like
¼ cup grade B maple syrup
1 tsp. vanilla extract
½ cup almond flour
½ cup + 1 Tbs coconut flour
½ tsp. baking soda
pinch of sea salt
1 cup dark chocolate chips
½ cup unsweetened coconut flakes

What to do
Preheat the oven to 350° F.
Combine the first 6 ingredients (eggs, coconut milk, coconut butter, coffee, maple syrup, and vanilla) in a bowl. Mix them together. I always use my favorite kitchen tool, my stick blender, to do the mixing.
In a separate bowl, combine the almond flour, coconut flour, baking soda, and salt. Stir.
Add the liquid, a little at a time, to the dry ingredients, mashing and stirring the mixture until smooth. Then, add half the chocolate chips to the mixture and stir them in.
Pour/push the mixture into the greased baking dish, smoothing it out with a spatula.
Top with coconut flakes, then chocolate chips.
Bake for 35 minutes, then allow it to cool.

Paleo Diet Recipes 365 Days of Paleo and Coconut Recipes by Mercedes Del Rey

308. Grain Free Steamed Christmas Puddings – GAPS & Paleo Friendly

Ingredients
150g sultanas
80g dried sour cherries or dried unsweetened cranberries, plus extra for garnish
100g currants
30g activated or raw almonds, roughly chopped
200g kombucha or freshly squeezed orange juice
zest of 1 orange
40g blanched almond meal
20g coconut flour
1/4 tsp nutmeg
1/2 tsp mixed spice
1/4 tsp cinnamon
55g tallow or coconut oil
40g apple, peeled & cored
2 eggs
1/4 tsp fine salt
1/4 tsp bicarb soda

Instructions
Weigh dried fruit and almonds into the Thermomix bowl, and add kombucha or orange juice.
Cook 6 mins/80C/reverse/speed soft. Remove to a large bowl and set aside to cool.
Place orange zest into clean, dry Thermomix bowl and chop 20 sec/speed 10.
Add almond meal, coconut flour, spices, salt, soda, apple, eggs and tallow or coconut oil into Thermomix bowl and mix 5 sec/speed 5. Scrape down sides of bowl.
Add soaked fruit and nuts back to bowl and mix 10 sec/reverse/speed 3.
Scoop mixture into silicone cupcake cups or small ramekins and place into the Varoma dish and tray, with lid on. Cups/ramekins should be about 3/4 full.
Place 500g water into Thermomix bowl and place Varoma in position. Cook 25 mins/Varoma/speed 2.
Allow puddings to cool, covered, and store in fridge until needed.
Drizzle with Coconut Vanilla Custard, with a dried cranberry or sour cherry on top for decoration.
Notes
I use my Thermomix to make these puddings - if you don't have a Thermomix, chop by hand, cook fruit gently on stovetop, and mix in remaining ingredients. Steam in a steamer or use traditional Christmas pudding cooking method.

Paleo Diet Recipes 365 Days of Paleo and Coconut Recipes by Mercedes Del Rey

309. Paleo Antioxidant Berry Shake

Ingredients
1/2 cup coconut milk
1/4 cup cold water
1/2 frozen banana
1/2 cup frozen raspberries
1/2 cup frozen blueberries
1 tbsp chia seeds
Directions
In a large cup (if using an immersion blender) or a blender, combine ingredients and blend until smooth. Add more water if necessary to reach desired consistency. Serve immediately.
Notes
Servings: 1
Difficulty: Easy

310. Perfect Paleo Loaf

Makes 1 traditional loaf
Ingredients:
- 1/2 cup + 2 tbsp coconut flour, sifted
- 2 tbsp finely ground golden flaxseed
- 1 tsp baking soda
- 6 eggs, separated
- 4 tbsp coconut oil, melted
- 1/2 cup coconut milk
- 1 tsp apple cider vinegar or lemon juice
- Low sodium salt (to taste)

Instruction:
1. Preheat your oven to 375 degrees F. Line a loaf pan with a sheet of parchment paper on it, brush some butter on the remaining uncovered sides.
2. In a large mixing bowl, sift together all dry ingredients; make sure all lumps are smoothed out.
3. Separate eggs, adding the yolks to the flour mixture and set aside the whites to a medium mixing bowl.
4. Add the melted coconut oil, coconut milk, and apple cider vinegar/lemon juice to the flour, mixing thoroughly. Expect the mixture to be dene and dry.
5. Whip egg whites with hand mixer until stiff peaks begin to form.
6. Fold egg whites into batter.
7. Spoon bread batter into a greased loaf pan. Smooth out the top with a spatula so that bread will bake evenly.
8. Bake for 35-40 minutes, covering bread with foil the last 5-10 minutes of baking.
9. Allow bread to cool for 5-10 minutes before transferring the bread to a cooling rack.
10. Slice and serve. Store any remaining bread in the refrigerator for up to 4 days.

Tips

It is very important to sift the coconut flour to remove any lumps, as it is a very dense flour.

Golden flaxseed as it adds a nice color to the bread making it look like a "multi-grain."

Whipping the egg whites allows the bread to be more fluffy and "slice-able."

This bread is not sweet. Many bread recipes have added honey or sweeteners, but if you want it to be a bit sweet, you can add a few drops of stevia.

311. Raw Pineapple Coconut Vegan Cheesecake

Crust:
4 dates, soaked until very soft1 cup dried organic, unsweetened coconut
Place soften dates and coconut in food processor and process until well blended.Pat into the bottom of an oiled 7 1/2 inch spring form pan.
 Filling:
2 1/2 cups young Thai coconut flesh (about 5 young coconuts)1/4 cup coconut water (from the coconuts)1/3 cup raw agave nectar or liquid sweetener of choice1 cup coconut oil, softened2 cups fresh pineapple chunks, separated
In high-speed blender, pureé the coconut flesh and coconut water together until smooth.Add the agave, coconut oil. You want this to be quite smooth so blend away until it is.Add 1 cup of the pineapple chunks. Blend until incorporated.Pulse the remaining pineapple chunks in the food processor until well chopped. Drain.Stir the pineapple into the coconut mixture, pour over crust and let set up in the refrigerator for 4 hours. Move to freezer and leave until firm.

312. Nutritious Paleo Tortillas

Ingredients
1/4 cup coconut flour (40 g)
1/4 teaspoon baking powder
8 egg whites (240 g or 1 cup)
1/2 cup water
A pinch of low sodium salt
coconut oil (as needed, for greasing the press or pan)
Instructions
1. In a bowl mix all ingredients. Set aside for five minutes. The batter takes about that long to hydrate and thicken.
*If necessary grease your tortilla press or pan with coconut oil.
Make the tortillas:
1. In a preheated electric tortilla press: Pour about a little less than 1/4 cup of batter onto the tortilla press. Quickly smooth out using a heat resistant spoon, and press the top of the press down to distribute the rest of the batter. Cook until the indicator on the press goes off.
2. In a pan over medium heat: Pour a little less than 1/4 cup of batter onto the pan. Quickly smooth out using a heat resistant spoon. Cook for 1 to 2 minutes or until the edges of the tortilla start to turn golden brown. Then flip and cook for an additional minute or two.
3. Transfer tortillas to a plate and cover with a paper towel to keep warm.
4. Serve with desired toppings and do your best to keep away from within hungry doggy mouths.

313. Perfect Paleo Bananacado Fudge Cupcakes

Ingredients
2 1/2 c. almond butter
1 1/4 c. stevia (or you can lower this to 3/4 c. and add an additional banana)
2 lg ripe bananas
3 medium avocados
3 eggs, beaten
3/4 c. cocoa powder
1 tbsp. vanilla
1 tsp baking soda
2 tsp baking powder

Instructions
In a large bowl, mix the almond butter and stevia.
In a blender or mixer, beat the eggs, banana, vanilla, cocoa powder and avocado to form a mousse-like consistency.
Add baking soda and baking powder.
Fold into the almond butter to make batter.
Pour into mini-cupcake tin (use the paper, it really makes a difference)
Bake at 350 for 15-18 minutes depending on size and desired consistency.

314. Paleo Sticky Date Pudding Cupcakes

Ingredients
For the muffins
Coconut Butter grease the muffin tray with
10 tbsp water
12 dates
1 ½ ripe banana, peeled and roughly chopped
2 ½ -3 tbsp coconut flour
1 tbsp vanilla extract or essence or 1 fresh vanilla bean, seeds scraped out
2 eggs
5 drops stevia liquid (May need a few more – please taste test)
½ tsp baking powder
For the sticky date ganache
5-6 dates, chopped
½ of orange, juice only
3 tbsp almond milk (coconut milk or water can also be used)
1 tsp vanilla extract or essence
2 drops stevia
Fresh raspberries or strawberries for garnish

Instructions
Preheat oven to 185°C (365 °F).
Grease muffin tins with the butter and set aside.
Heat the dates and water in a small saucepan over low heat until the dates break down and thicken. Use a fork to mash them together and set aside.
Place the coconut flour, egg, banana, vanilla extract and baking powder in a blender or food processor and mix well until well combined and aerated.
Add the dates to the banana mixture and combine. Evenly distribute into the ramekins. Cook in the oven for about 20-22 minutes.
While the muffins are in the oven, place the sticky date ganache ingredients in a small saucepan over a low heat and cook for about 3-4 minutes or until the dates break down. Mash with a fork and whisk until thickened. Set aside.
Allow the muffins to rest for 5 minutes before removing them to a serving plate. Scoop a dollop of sticky date ganache paste on top and garnish with a few raspberries.

315. Vanilla Paleo Cupcakes

Ingredients:
Apple Cakes:
4 tablespoons (or ¼ cup) of Grass-Fed/Clarified Butter or Extra Virgin Coconut Oil
½ cup Unsweetened Applesauce
4 Eggs
1 teaspoon Vanilla Extract
5 drops stevia liquid (May need a few more – please taste test)
¾ cup Almond Flour
2 teaspoons Cinnamon
½ teaspoon Baking Powder
1/8 teaspoon low sodium Salt

Cinnamon Frosting:
1 cup room temperature coconut oil
5 drops stevia liquid (May need a few more – please taste test)
1 teaspoon Vanilla Extract
4 tablespoons (or ¼ cup) Arrowroot
2 teaspoons Coconut Flour
2 teaspoons Cinnamon
2 tablespoons Chilled Coconut Milk Cream

Topping:
½ Apple Thinly Sliced
Cinnamon for Dusting

Instructions
Apple Cakes:
Preheat oven to 350 degrees F. Line mini cupcake pan with 24 paper liners.
Melt the butter then whisk in with the applesauce, eggs, vanilla, and stevia.
Add the almond flour, cinnamon, baking powder, and salt to the wet ingredients and mix until evenly combined.
Evenly distribute into the 24 mini cupcake liners {about 1 tablespoon of batter each} and bake at 350 F for 18 – 19 minutes. The cakes are done when a toothpick can be poked in and come out without any batter on the stick.
Let the cool completely.

Cinnamon Frosting:
Whisk the shortening, stevia, vanilla, arrowroot, coconut flour, and cinnamon together until smooth.
Add the chilled coconut milk cream and whisk again until smooth.
Use immediately. Either spoon the frosting into a gallon plastic bag or a pastry bag.
Gently frost each cupcake with your desired amount of frosting.
Store the rest of the frosting in the refrigerator. Let it come to room temperature before you use as frosting again.
Topping:
Top each cupcake with a thin slice of fresh green apple and dust with ground cinnamon.
If you don't enjoy the cupcakes immediately, store them in an airtight container in the refrigerator.

316. Paleo Vanilla Cupcakes

Serves: 6 cupcakes
Ingredients
¼ cup coconut flour
⅛ teaspoon celtic sea salt
⅛ teaspoon baking soda
3 large eggs
¼ cup room temperature coconut oil
5 drops stevia liquid (May need a few more – please taste test)
1 tablespoon vanilla extract
Instructions
In a food processor, combine coconut flour, salt and baking soda
Pulse in eggs, shortening, honey and vanilla
Line a cupcake pan with 6 paper liners and scoop ¼ cup into each
Bake at 350° for 20-24 minutes
Cool for 1 hour
Frost with Paleo Chocolate Frosting
Serve

Paleo Diet Recipes 365 Days of Paleo and Coconut Recipes by Mercedes Del Rey

317. Paleo Chocolate Cupcake with "Peanut Butter" Frosting

Ingredients
Cake Ingredients
1/4 cup coconut flour
3 large eggs
1/4 cup cup unsweetened cacao powder
1/3 cup raw honey
1/4 cup coconut oil
1/2 tsp baking soda
1 tsp vanilla
Pinch of salt
Frosting Ingredients
3/4 cup sunflower butter
3/4 cup Tropical Traditions Palm Shortening –or– 3/4 cup organic butter
1/3 cup raw honey
2 tsp vanilla
pinch salt
Instructions
Make your frosting first
Frosting Instructions
Using a stand mixer or hand mixer, combine sunflower butter and shortening on medium-high speed until fluffy. Takes about 3 minutes.
Add honey, vanilla and pinch of salt. Whip on high for another couple of minutes.
It should look like frosting, thick enough to spread on a cupcake.
Place in fridge while you bake your cupcakes
Cake Instructions
Combine dry ingredients together in a bowl: coconut flour, cacao powder, baking soda, salt
Whisk eggs in another small bowl and add melted coconut oil, honey and vanilla
Combine with dry ingredients and mix
Pour into muffin cups of your choice
Bake at 350º F for 15-18 min.
Makes about 6-8 cupcakes
Once cooled, frost those yummy cakes!
We sprinkled on a few mini dark chocolate chips just for fun :)
Frosting holds up well, but refrigerate if you don't eat them all right away.

318. Addictive & Healthy Paleo Nachos

Ingredients

- 2 medium tomatoes, diced and seeded
- 2 tbsp fresh cilantro, chopped
- 1-2 tbsp lime juice
- 2 cups guacamole
- 2 tbsp green onions, chopped

For the sweet potato chips
- 3 large sweet potatoes
- 3 tbsp melted coconut oil
- 1 tsp salt

For the meat
- 1 medium yellow onion, finely diced
- 1 tbsp coconut oil
- 1 green chili, diced
- 1 lb. ground beef
- 2 cloves garlic, minced
- 1 tsp smoked paprika
- 1/2 tsp ground cumin
- 1 tbsp tomato paste
- 12 oz. canned diced tomatoes
- 1 tsp salt
- 1/2 tsp pepper

Instructions

To make the sweet potato chips, preheat the oven to 375 degrees F. Peel the sweet potatoes and slice thinly, using either a mandolin or sharp knife. In a large bowl, toss them with coconut oil and salt. Place the chips in a single layer on a rimmed baking sheet covered with parchment paper. Bake in the oven for 10 minutes, then flip the chips over and bake for another 10 minutes. For the last ten minutes, watch the chips closely and pull off any chips that start to brown, until all of the chips are cooked.

While the potato chips are baking, start preparing the beef. Melt the coconut oil in a large skillet over medium heat. Add the onion and chili to the pan and sauté for 3-4 minutes until softened. Add the ground beef and cook for 4-5 minutes, stirring regularly. Add the garlic, diced tomatoes, tomato paste, and remaining spices and stir well to combine. Bring the mixture to a simmer and then turn the heat down to medium-low. Cook, covered, for 20-25 minutes, stirring regularly.

Stir the chopped tomatoes, lime juice, and cilantro into the beef mixture. Adjust salt and pepper to taste. Remove from heat.

To assemble the nachos, form a large circle with the sweet potato chips on a platter. Add the beef mixture into the middle of the circle, and then top with guacamole and green onions.

Notes

Servings: 4-6
Difficulty: Medium

319. Homemade Paleo Tortilla Chips

Ingredients
1 cup almond flour
1 egg white
1/2 tsp salt
1/2 tsp chili powder
1/2 tsp garlic powder
1/2 tsp cumin
1/4 tsp onion powder
1/4 tsp paprika

Directions
Preheat the oven to 325 degrees F. In a large bowl, combine all of the ingredients together until they form an even dough. Roll out the dough between two pieces of parchment paper, as thinly as possible. Remove the top layer of parchment paper. Cut the dough into desired shapes for chips.

Move the dough, with the parchment paper, onto a baking sheet. Bake for 11-13 minutes, until golden brown. Remove from the oven and let cool 5 minutes. Use a spatula to remove the chips from the paper. Serve with guacamole or salsa.

320. Paleo Chocolate Cookies (I Can't Get Enough of These)

Ingredients
2 tbsp and 2 tsp coconut oil
3 oz. unsweetened dark chocolate
1/4 cup honey
2 eggs
1 1/2 tsp vanilla extract
1/2 cup coconut flour
1/2 tsp cinnamon

Instructions

In a large microwave-safe bowl, melt the coconut oil and chocolate in the microwave, stirring intermittently. Let cool for 5 minutes.

Add the eggs, vanilla, and honey to the chocolate mixture. Stir well to make sure not to scramble the eggs. Add in the coconut flour and cinnamon and mix well. Place in the refrigerator for approximately 30 minutes, until slightly hardened.

Preheat oven to 350 degrees F. Roll out the dough between two pieces of parchment paper until 1/4-inch thick. Cut out shapes with a cookie cutter and carefully place on a parchment-lined baking sheet. Repeat this step for remaining dough. Bake cookies for 12-15 minutes. Allow to cool before serving.

Notes
Servings: approximately 18 cookies
Difficulty: Medium

321. Easy Paleo Shepherd's Pie

For the top layer
1 large head cauliflower, cut into florets
2 tbsp ghee, melted
1 tsp spicy Paleo mustard
Salt and freshly ground black pepper, to taste
Fresh parsley, to garnish
For the bottom layer
1 tbsp coconut oil
1/2 large onion, diced
3 carrots, diced
2 celery stalks, diced
1 lb. lean ground beef
2 tbsp tomato paste
1 cup chicken broth
1 tsp dry mustard
1/4 tsp cinnamon
1/8 tsp ground clove
Salt and freshly ground black pepper, to taste

Instructions

Place a couple inches of water in a large pot. Once the water is boiling, place steamer insert and then cauliflower florets into the pot and cover. Steam for 12-14 minutes, until tender. Drain and return cauliflower to the pot.

Add the ghee, mustard, salt, and pepper to the cauliflower. Using an immersion blender or food processor, combine the ingredients until smooth. Set aside.

Meanwhile, heat the coconut oil in a large skillet over medium heat. Add the onion, celery, and carrots and sauté for 5 minutes. Add in the ground beef and cook until browned.

Stir the tomato paste, chicken broth, and remaining spices into the meat mixture. Season to taste with salt and pepper. Simmer until most of the liquid has evaporated, about 8 minutes, stirring occasionally.

Distribute the meat mixture evenly among four ramekins and spread the pureed cauliflower on top. Use a fork to create texture in the cauliflower and drizzle with olive oil. Place under the broiler for 5-7 minutes until the top turns golden. Sprinkle with fresh parsley and serve.

Notes
Servings: 4
Difficulty: Medium

322. Paleo Apple Pie Cupcakes with Cinnamon Frosting

Ingredients:
WET INGREDIENTS
- 5 Eggs, room temperature
- 1/2 cup applesauce (you can make your own or use a sugar-free pre-made brand)
- 1/2 cup raw honey, melted
- 1/3 cupcoconut oil, melted

DRY INGREDIENTS
- 1 1/4 cup finely ground blanch almond flour
- 1/2 cup coconut flour
- 1/2 tsp. sea salt
- 1/2 tsp. baking powder

FROSTING INGREDIENTS:
- 1 cupcoconut oil
- 3 Tbsp. raw honey
- 2 tsp. cinnamon
- Dash sea salt

Equipment:
- Muffin tin
- 12 baking cups
- 2 medium mixing bowls
Hand mixe
- For

Directions:
1. Preheat oven to 350F. Line muffin pan with baking cups.
2. Combine all wet ingredients in a medium sized mixing bowl. Beat on medium with a hand mixer for about 30 seconds.
3. Combine all dry ingredients in another medium sized bowl. Mix together with a fork to break apart any clumps.
4. Add the dry ingredients to the wet ingredients and beat for about 20 seconds. Make sure all ingredients are combined.
5. Fill each lined muffin tin about 3/4 of the way full. Bake for 25-30 minutes or until a toothpick comes out clean in the center.
6. Take the cupcakes out of the oven and set aside to cool completely. All the way cooled! But feel free to sneak one to nibble on while the rest cool off.
7. Once the cupcakes have cooled, make the frosting! Combine all of the ingredients into a medium mixing bowl and beat on medium speed for about 30 seconds until well combines. Ice those cupcakes and get to eating!

323. Paleo French Toast with Blueberry Syrup

Ingredients
1 loaf Paleo bread (I used this recipe for Paleo Bread)
1/2 cup almond milk
2 eggs
1/2 tbsp vanilla
1 tsp cinnamon
Instructions
In a large bowl, whisk together the coconut milk, eggs, vanilla and cinnamon.
Heat a griddle or non-stick skillet to medium-high. Coat pan with coconut oil. Dip a slice of bread into the batter mixture to coat both sides, letting any excess drip off. Place the bread onto the pan and cook each side until slightly browned. Repeat with remaining bread. Serve warm.
Notes
Servings: 4
Difficulty: Easy

324. The Best Paleo Brownies (Chocolaty Goodness)

Ingredients
1 cup paleo-friendly almond butter
1/3 cup maple syrup
1 egg
2 tbsp ghee
1 tsp vanilla
1/3 cup cocoa powder
1/2 tsp baking soda
Instructions
Preheat the oven to 325 degrees F. In a large bowl, whisk together the almond butter, syrup, egg, ghee, and vanilla. Stir in the cocoa powder and baking soda.
Pour the batter into a 9-inch baking pan. Bake for 20-23 minutes, until the brownie is done, but still soft in the middle.
Notes
Servings: 6
Difficulty: Easy

325. Paleo Chocolate Cranberry Muffins

INGREDIENTS
200 grams almond flour (about 2 cups)
⅓ cup cacao powder
2 tablespoons coconut sugar
½ teaspoon baking soda
⅛ teaspoon salt
3 eggs
¼ cup honey
¼ cup ghee, melted
1 teaspoon vanilla extract
1 teaspoon apple cider vinegar
½ cup cranberries, thawed if frozen

INSTRUCTIONS
Preheat oven to 325 degrees and grease or line muffin tin.
Combine almond flour, cacao, coconut sugar, baking soda, and salt in a large bowl. Combine eggs, honey, ghee, vanilla, and apple cider vinegar in medium bowl. Stir wet ingredients into dry ingredients, then fold in cranberries.
Using a large ice cream or cookie scoop, fill muffin cups ¾ full.
Bake 20 - 25 minutes, until toothpick inserted in center comes out clean.

326. Salt and Vinegar Zucchini Chips

Ingredients
4 cups thinly sliced zucchini (about 2-3 medium)
2 tablespoons extra virgin olive oil
2 tablespoons white balsamic vinegar
2 teaspoons coarse sea salt
Instructions
Use a mandolin or slice zucchini as thin as possible.
In a small bowl whisk olive oil and vinegar together.
Place zucchini in a large bowl and toss with oil and vinegar.
Add zucchini in even layers to dehydrator then sprinkle with coarse sea salt.
Depending on how thin you sliced the zucchini and on your dehydrator the drying time will vary, anywhere from 8-14 hours.
To make in the oven: Line a cookie sheet with parchment paper. Lay zucchini evenly. Bake at 200 degrees F for 2-3 hours. Rotate half way during cooking time.
Store chips in an airtight container.

Paleo Diet Recipes 365 Days of Paleo and Coconut Recipes by Mercedes Del Rey

327. Nutritious Paleo Tortillas

Ingredients
1/4 cup coconut flour (40 g)
1/4 teaspoon baking powder
8 egg whites (240 g or 1 cup)
1/2 cup water
A pinch of low sodium salt
coconut oil (as needed, for greasing the press or pan)

Instructions
1. In a bowl mix all ingredients. Set aside for five minutes. The batter takes about that long to hydrate and thicken.
*If necessary grease your tortilla press or pan with coconut oil.
Make the tortillas:
1. In a preheated electric tortilla press: Pour about a little less than 1/4 cup of batter onto the tortilla press. Quickly smooth out using a heat resistant spoon, and press the top of the press down to distribute the rest of the batter. Cook until the indicator on the press goes off.
2. In a pan over medium heat: Pour a little less than 1/4 cup of batter onto the pan. Quickly smooth out using a heat resistant spoon. Cook for 1 to 2 minutes or until the edges of the tortilla start to turn golden brown. Then flip and cook for an additional minute or two.
3. Transfer tortillas to a plate and cover with a paper towel to keep warm.
4. Serve with desired toppings and do your best to keep away from within hungry doggy mouths.

328. Perfect Paleo Bananacado Fudge Cupcakes

Ingredients
2 1/2 c. almond butter
1 1/4 c. stevia (or you can lower this to 3/4 c. and add an additional banana)
2 lg ripe bananas
3 medium avocados
3 eggs, beaten
3/4 c. cocoa powder
1 tbsp. vanilla
1 tsp baking soda
2 tsp baking powder

Instructions
In a large bowl, mix the almond butter and stevia.
In a blender or mixer, beat the eggs, banana, vanilla, cocoa powder and avocado to form a mousse-like consistency.
Add baking soda and baking powder.
Fold into the almond butter to make batter.
Pour into mini-cupcake tin (use the paper, it really makes a difference)
Bake at 350 for 15-18 minutes depending on size and desired consistency.

329. Incredibly Easy Paleo Chicken Soup

Ingredients
4 cups (946 mL) chicken broth
2 inch (5.1 cm) piece fresh ginger, sliced into thin coins
1 inch piece (2.5 cm) fresh turmeric*, sliced into thin coins
3 cloves garlic, peeled & smashed
½ teaspoon (3 mL) fish sauce
2 cups (280 g) cooked shredded chicken
4 ounces (113 g) shiitake mushrooms, sliced
3 green onions (48 g), white and light green parts, thinly sliced
1 medium carrot (40 g), julienned or shredded
Sea salt, to taste
Optional: 1 cup (227 g) zucchini noodles, kelp noodles, or mountain yam shiritaki noodles
Optional: Paleo Sriracha for drizzling
Instructions

Pour the chicken broth into a medium pot, and add the ginger, turmeric, garlic and fish sauce. Bring to a boil, then reduce to a simmer for 20 to 30 minutes to really infuse the broth with flavor. Note: If using turmeric powder (ground turmeric), start with ¼ teaspoon (0.5 gram), and increase to ½ teaspoon (1 gram), depending on your preference. I find turmeric powder to be insanely potent, much more so than the fresh root, so always add less and bump it up if you'd like. While the broth is simmering, prepare the rest of the ingredients.

Using a slotted spoon, remove the ginger, turmeric and garlic. Discard. Or, if you like to live dangerously, leave it all in the soup and pick around it while you're eating (like I did in the photo). Just be aware: Biting into a large chunk of ginger, turmeric or garlic is usually not pleasant.

Add the chicken, mushrooms, green onions, carrot and if desired, your noodles. Heat about 5 minutes on medium-low or until everything is warmed through. Taste and adjust the seasoning with sea salt.

Serve with a drizzle of sriracha for some extra heat.

Notes
*If you can't find fresh turmeric root, sub in ¼ teaspoon (0.5 g) turmeric powder. When working with any form of turmeric, take care because it stains hands, clothing and porous surfaces.

330. Paleo Chicken Soup

Ingredients:
2 pounds uncooked chicken breasts/thighs
1 pound diced carrots
2 medium sweet potatoes cubed (I love white sweet potatoes!) or 1 pound parsnips diced
6 ribs/stalks celery chopped
1 onion diced
2-3 garlic cloves diced finely
2 to 3 tsp sea salt
1/2 to 1 tsp black pepper
4 cups chopped kale or collards.
6 to 8 cups Chicken Broth/Stock
Optional: 1 to 2 tbsp dried herbs (rosemary, thyme, sage)
Directions:
Grab your slow cooker or giant stock pot. Add all of ingredients except for the broth.
If you like a thicker soup, add just enough broth to barely cover the ingredients. If you enjoy a more broth-y soup add the full amount of broth.
Slow Cooker: 7 to 8 hours on low, 3-4 hours on high. Stovetop: Bring the soup to a boil, cover, and reduce to simmer (low) – leave for one hour.
Once the soup is finished cooking (chicken is cooked through and veggies are soft) remove the chicken and shred or chop it.

Paleo Diet Recipes 365 Days of Paleo and Coconut Recipes by Mercedes Del Rey

331. Paleo Chicken Soup with Nuddles

Ingredients
2 tablespoons coconut oil
1 onion, minced
1 carrot, peeled and sliced thin
1 rib celery, sliced
2 teaspoons minced fresh thyme or 1/2 teaspoon dried
2 1/2 quarts homemade bone broth
3 cups shredded chicken
1/4 cup minced fresh parsley
3-4 eggs, lightly beaten
sea salt and pepper to taste

Instructions
1. Heat the oil in a large Dutch oven over medium-high heat until shimmering. Add the onion, carrot, and celery and cook until softened, 3-4 minutes. Stir in the thyme, bone broth, and chicken. Bring to a simmer and cook until the vegetables are tender, about 15 minutes. Stir in parsley.
2. Stir soup gently so that it is moving in a circle. Pour beaten eggs into soup in a slow steady stream. This will create "noodles" for the soup. Remove soup from heat and let stand for 2 minutes. Break up the eggs using a fork. Season with sea salt and pepper to taste before serving.

332. PALEO CROCK POT CHICKEN SOUP

Ingredients
1 medium onion, chopped
3 celery stalks, diced
3 carrots, diced
1 teaspoon apple cider vinegar
1 tablespoon herbes de Provence, or several sprigs fresh herbs
2 organic chicken breasts, bone-in, skin-on
2 organic chicken thighs, bone-in, skin-on
1 teaspoon sea salt
½ teaspoon fresh ground pepper
3-4 cups filtered water

Instructions
Layer all ingredients in crock pot in order listed, making sure chicken is bone side down on top of vegetables. Add enough water to cover vegetables and come half way up chicken, between 3 and 4 cups.
Cook on low for 6-8 hours.
Remove chicken and let cool slightly. Remove skin and bones. Shred chicken meat and add back to soup in crock pot. Adjust seasonings, reheat, and serve.

333. Paleo Stuffed Breakfast Peppers

Ingredients
2 bell peppers – your choice of colour
4 eggs
1 cup white mushrooms
1 cup broccoli
¼ tsp cayenne pepper
Salt and pepper, to taste

Directions
Preheat oven to 375 degrees Fahrenheit.
Dice up your vegetables of choice.
In a medium sized bowl, mix eggs, salt, pepper, cayenne pepper, and vegetables.
Cut peppers into equal halves. A tip: Try to buy peppers that are symmetrical and have somewhat flat sides – this makes it easier for them to balance while baking.
Core the peppers so that they're clean enough to add the filling.
Pour a quarter of the egg / vegetable mix into each pepper half, adding more vegetables to the top to fill in any empty space.
Place on baking sheet and cook approximately 35 minutes or until eggs are cooked to your liking.
Serve and enjoy! I personally like mine with a dash of hot sauce on top.

Notes
This recipe makes 2 servings.
Nutrition Facts Per Serving
Calories: 186
Total Fat: 9.4g
Saturated Fat: 2.8g
Carbs: 12.1g
Fiber: 4.0g
Protein: 14.6g

334. Blushing Beet Salad

Ingredients:
2 large beets, washed and stems cut off
1 cup carrots, peeled and cooked
1 tbsp cilantro, chopped
1 tbsp diced onion
2 tbsp paleo mayonnaise
Low sodium salt and pepper
Instructions:
Boil beets in water until soft, about 50 minutes. Peel and cut into small 1/2" cubes. Cook carrots until tender and cut into bite size cubes. Combine diced onion, carrots, beets, mayonnaise, cilantro, low sodium salt and pepper.

335. Cheeky Chicken Salad

Ingredients:
olive oil spray
2 tsp olive oil
16 oz (2 large) skinless boneless chicken breasts, cut into 24 1-inch chunks
Low sodium salt and pepper to taste
4 cups shredded romaine
1 cup shredded red cabbage
For the Skinny Cheeky Sauce:
2 1/2 tbsppaleo mayonnaise
2 tbsp scallions, chopped fine plus more for topping
1 1/2 tsp chilli flakes
Instructions:
Preheat oven to 425°F. Spray a baking sheet with olive oil spray.

Season chicken with low sodium salt and pepper, olive oil and mix well so the olive oil evenly coats all of the chicken.

Meanwhile combine the sauce in a medium bowl. When the chicken is ready, drizzle it over the top and enjoy!!

336. Melting Mustard Chicken

Ingredients:
8 small chicken thighs, skin removed
3 tsp mustard powder
1 tbsp paleo mayonnaise
1 clove garlic, crushed
1 lime, squeezed, and lime zest
3/4 tsp pepper
Low sodium salt
dried parsley

Instructions:

Preheat oven to 400°. Rinse the chicken and remove the skin and all fat. Pat dry …place in a large bowl and season generously with low sodium salt. In a small bowl combine mustard, mayonnaise, lime juice, lime zest, garlic and pepper. Mix well. Pour over chicken, tossing well to coat.

Spray a large baking pan with a little Pam to prevent sticking since all the fat and skin was removed from chicken. Place chicken to fit in a single layer.

Top the chicken with dried parsley. Bake until cooked through, about 30-35 minutes.

Finish the chicken under the broiler until it is golden brown. Serve chicken with the pan juices drizzled over the top.

337. Easy Paleo Spaghetti Squash & Meatballs

Ingredients
One medium spaghetti squash.
One pound of ground Italian sausage.
One can of tomato sauce, I used a 14 ounce can.
2 tbsp of hot pepper relish (optional).
4 to 6 cloves of garlic, whole.
2 tbsp of olive oil.
Italian seasoning (Oregano, Basil, Thyme) to taste, I used about 2 tsp

Instruction
Make sure you use a large 6 quart slow cooker for this recipe.
Dump your tomato sauce, olive oil, garlic, hot pepper relish and Italian seasoning into your slow cooker and stir well.
Cut your squash in half and scoop out the seeds.
Place your 2 squash halves face down into your slow cooker.
Roll your ground sausage into meatballs, then fit as many as you can in the sauce around the squash. I was able to work in about a half pound worth.
Cook on High for 3 hours or cook on low for 5 hours.
Use a large fork to pull the "spaghetti" out of your squash, then top with your meatballs and sauce.
Garnish with parsley if you feel fancy, and enjoy!

338. Paleo Pulled Pork Sliders

Ingredients
1. Large pork roast
2. 1 large onion, sliced
3. 3 minced garlic cloves
4. 2 tsp cumin
5. 2 tsp chili powder
6. 1 tsp pepper
7. 2 tsp oregano
8. 1 tsp paprika
9. 1/2 tsp cayenne pepper
10. 1/2 tsp cinnamon
11. 2 tsp sea salt
12. juice of 1 lime
13. juice of 1 lemon

Instructions
1. Stir together the spices and rub all over the roast. Lay the onion slices down on the bottom of the slow cooker, and squeeze half of the fruit juices in. Put the roast in the crockpot and squeeze the remaining lime and lemon juice over it. Cook on low overnight or throughout the day about 8 hours (you really can't overcook it to be honest). When done, shred it with two forks until it's completely 'pulled'.

The "Buns"
1. 1 large sweet potato (try to go for a nice evenly round one, remember the diameter will be the size of your sliders)
2. 2 tbsp coconut oil
3. 1/4 tsp cumin
4. 1/4 tsp paprika
5. dash of sea salt

Instructions
1. Slice the sweet potato into 1/4" thick rounds. Lay them out on a parchment paper-lined cookie sheet.
2. Brush each slice with coconut oil and sprinkle with the spices, then flip and do the same on the other side.
3. Bake at 425 degrees Farenheit for 35 minutes until golden brown on the outside and cooked all the way through, flipping halfway through. You may need to crank it up to 450 if your oven isn't nice and sizzly.
4. Top a patty with pulled pork, and add any other toppings or sauces you'd like (I just used some lettuce from our garden).
5. Finish with the top patty and enjoy your delightful little sliders!

339. Basic Balsamic Steak Marinade

Ingredients
1 lb. flank steak
Salt and pepper
2 cloves garlic, minced
1/2 tbsp oregano
1/2 tbsp rosemary
1 tsp Paleo mustard
1/4 cup balsamic vinegar
1 tsp honey
1/2 cup extra virgin olive oil

Instructions

Stir together the garlic, oregano, rosemary, mustard, vinegar, honey, and olive oil.

Salt and pepper the steak and place in a shallow dish, then pour the marinade over the steak. Cover and place in the refrigerator for 3-12 hours.

To cook the steak, heat the grill to medium and cook each side approximately 4-5 minutes, or until desired doneness. Let stand for about 5 minutes before slicing and serving.

Notes
Servings: 3
Difficulty: Medium

340. Lemon Tilapia Ajillo

Ingredients:
6 (6 oz each) tilapia filets
4 cloves garlic, crushed
2 tbsp olive oil
2 tbsp fresh lemon juice
4 tsp fresh parsley
Low sodium salt and pepper
cooking spray
large romaine lettuce, 1 grated carrot, half grated onion, handful baby tomatoes
Basic Paleo Dressing:
2 tblspoon best quality olive oil
1 tbspn apple cider vinegar
Squirt of fresh lemon juice
Half teaspoon garlic powder and half teaspoon onion powder
Black pepper to taste
Instructions:
Preheat oven to 400°.
Melt butter on a low flame in a small sauce pan. Add garlic and saute on low for about 1 minute. Add the lemon juice and shut off flame.
Spray the bottom of a baking dish lightly with cooking spray. Place the fish on top and season with low sodium salt and pepper. Pour the lemon butter mixture on the fish and top with fresh parsley. Bake at 400° until cooked, about 15 minutes.
Serve with a mixed salad and paleo dressing

Paleo Diet Recipes 365 Days of Paleo and Coconut Recipes by Mercedes Del Rey

341. Paleo crock Bone Broth

Ingredients
2 bags beef bones or 2 chicken carcasses
1 large onion, sliced in half
1 head garlic, sliced in half
3-‒4 slices celery, cut into 1" pieces
1 cup baby carrots
1 large handful fresh thyme or sage
1 tablespoon apple cider vinegar per pound of bones
Water

Instructions
Place all ingredients in a 5‒-7 quart slow cooker. Fill with enough water to completely immerse. Cover and cook for 12 hours on low.
Remove large bones with tongs, and pour the broth through a slotted spoon into freezer-safe containers or mason jars. Cool and freeze what you don't plan to use within 4 days. Frozen bone broth will last up to 6 months in the freezer. Enjoy!

342. Paleo Phobroth

Ingredients
1. 1 onion, halved
2. 2" fresh ginger, halved lengthwise
3. 1 teaspoon avocado oil
4. 6 cups of Bare Bones Beef Broth
5. 4 cups of filtered water
6. 2 tablespoons fish sauce
7. 1 teaspoon sea salt

Spices
1. 1 cinnamon stick
2. 6 whole star anise
3. 5 whole cloves
4. 2 cardamom pods
5. 1 tablespoon fennel seeds

Directions:
Wrap the above ingredients in cheesecloth and securely tie
1. 1.5 lbs. of sirloin, very thinly sliced
2. 3 to 4 large parsnips, peeled

Toppings
1. lime wedges
2. chilli peppers
3. basil
4. mint
5. cilantro
6. bean sprouts
7. hot sauce

coconut aminos

Char your ginger and onions, by placing them on a baking sheet in the highest position of your oven (toaster oven works great for this!). Turn your broiler on high. Brush the onions and ginger with avocado oil and place them on your baking sheet. Broil for 10 minutes and then turn and continue to broil for another 5 to 10 minutes.

In a large pot, add the broth, filtered water, the charred onions and ginger, fish sauce, salt and spices wrapped in cheesecloth. Cover the broth and bring to a light boil and then turn down to a simmer. Continue simmering for 1 to 1.5 hours.

Towards the end of your broth's cooking time, slice the parsnips and thinly slice the meat and set in the fridge, until ready to use.

Put the broth through a mesh strainer to remove the ginger, onions and spices. Return it to the pot. Taste the broth and adjust the seasoning. The broth is the star of the show, so make sure it tastes great. You can add more salt or fish sauce, if it is not salty enough. If it is too salty, you can even add a little bit of honey to balance it out.

Bring your broth back to a light boil. Add the sliced meat to the strained broth and allow it to cook through. This is how I do it. Some people place the meat in individual bowls and pour the piping hot broth over it. Which I think is the more traditional method, but I prefer to cook it all in the large pot.

Add parsnips to the bottom of each bowl, ladle hot piping broth and meat into each bowl. Garnish with your favourite toppings and enjoy!

343. Fantastic Paleo Broth

Ingredients
1 quart beef bone broth (see above notes)
1 piece ginger root
1 onion
1 beef steak thickly cut
2 whole star anise
1 tsp. fennel
1 tsp. coriander
2 whole cloves
1 stick cinnamon
1 cardamom pod
2 Tbsp. fish sauce I used the liquid that comes off from my homemade anchovies.
 Garnishes spicy peppers, lime slices, sprouts, basil leaves, etc.

Instructions
Begin by making your beef bone broth as explained above. You can either add in your spices during that process or separate out some broth and continue with the recipe as follows.
Simmer your broth in a pot on the stove with your spice blend added in. I usually put my spices into a cotton bag to make for easier straining later on. As you simmer the broth, skim off any foam that comes to the top.
Meanwhile, wash both your ginger root and your (peeled) onion, slice them in half, and place them on a baking sheet in your oven.
Broil them until they get dark on top.
Once your ginger and onion are ready, add them to your simmering broth to give it more flavour.
Keep simmering for around half an hour, or until the soup has absorbed the flavours of the spices to your liking. At this point, I like to add in the fish sauce to taste. I start by adding one tablespoon and then taste it and then add more, a little bit at a time, if I think it needs it.
Remove your broth from the stove and remove the ginger and onion. I like reserving the onion for adding back to the soup later on. Strain the broth if necessary to get out any of the remaining spices, and put the broth back into the pot.
Meanwhile, I like to sear the outside of the beef that I will be adding to the pho. Many people like to thinly slice it raw and add it to the soup that way. I prefer to sear the edges first, leaving it very rare inside.
When you are ready to serve the soup, add the broth to each bowl. Thinly slice the seared beef and place the thin slices on top of the soup. The heat of the soup will help lightly cook the thin slices.
Serve with garnishes that each person can add to their bowl of soup as desired.

344. Tasty Tomato Tilapia

Ingredients:
2 tbsp extra virgin olive oil
4 (6 oz) tilapia filets
2 garlic cloves, crushed
2 shallots, minced
2 tomatoes, chopped
2 tbsp capers
1/4 cup white wine
Low sodium salt and fresh pepper

Instructions:
Brush fish with 1 tbsp olive and season with low sodium salt and pepper.
In a medium sauté pan, heat remaining olive oil. Add garlic and shallots and sauté on medium-low about 4-5 minutes. Add tomatoes and season with low sodium salt and pepper. Add wine and sauté until wine reduces, about 5 minutes. Add capers and sauté an additional minute.
Meanwhile, set broiler to low and place fish about 8 inches from the flame. Broil until fish is cooked through, about 7 minutes.
Place fish on a platter and top with tomato caper sauce.
Eat with a green salad and paleo dressing

345. Beet Sprout Divine Salad

Ingredients:
1/2 pound Brussels sprouts, ends trimmed, outer leaves removed, and cut in half lengthwise
4 small red beets, tops trimmed to 1/2-inch, washed and cut in half lengthwise
4 tablespoons plus 1/3 cup extra virgin olive oil
1 tablespoon paleo Dijon mustard
Stevia to taste
Squeeze of lemon juice
Coarse low sodium salt
Grinding coarse black pepper
1 small red onion thinly sliced into rings
Instructions:
Preheat the oven to 350.
Pour 2 tablespoons olive oil in a baking dish. Toss the Brussels sprouts in the oil; sprinkle them with low sodium salt and pepper and roast them for 20 minutes.
Turn them once during the cooking. They are done when a small knife easily pierces them.
Pour 2 tablespoons of the olive oil on a sheet of aluminum foil and place
it on a baking sheet. Toss the beet halves in the olive oil. Sprinkle them with low sodium salt and pepper and, keeping them in a single layer, fold and seal the foil over them. Bake on the baking sheet until a knife easily pierces them.
When cool enough to handle, peel the beets and cut them into 1/4-inch slices.
Meanwhile combine the 1/3 cup olive oil, mustard, stevia, lemon juice and low sodium salt and pepper in a small bowl.
Toss the Ingredients, add the dressing and serve at room temperature.

346. Paleo Keto Bone Broth

Ingredients
3.3 lb oxtail (1.5 kg) or mixed with assorted bones (chicken feet, marrow bones, etc.)
2 medium carrots
1 medium parsnip or parsley root
2 medium celery stalks
1 medium white onion, skin on
5 cloves garlic, peeled
2 tbsp apple cider vinegar or fresh lemon juice
2-3 bay leaves
1 tbsp salt (I like pink Himalayan)
8-10 cups water, enough to cover the bones, no more than 2/3 capacity of your pressure cooker or 3/4 capacity of your Dutch oven or 3/4 capacity of your slow cooker

Instructions
Peel the root vegetables and cut them into thirds. Halve the onion and peel and halve the garlic cloves. Keeping the onion skin on will help the broth get a nice golden colour. Cut the celery into thirds. Place everything into the pressure cooker (or slow cooker) and add the bay leaves.

Add the oxtail and bones. You can use any bones you like: chicken, pork or beef, with or without meat. Because I used chicken and turkey bones with some skin on, the fat ended up being quite runny. You can still use it for cooking but I binned it.

Oxtail is rich in gelatin and contains more fat. Although traditional bone broth is made just from bones, especially beef marrowbones, I found oxtail to give the best flavor to my broth. The advantage of using oxtail is that it will yield 3 superfoods: bone broth, tender oxtail meat and tallow. Tallow is great when used for cooking the same way as ghee or lard.

Add 8-10 cups of water or up to 2/3 of your pressure cooker, slow cooker or Dutch oven, vinegar or freshly squeezed lemon juice and bay leaves. Make sure you use the vinegar or lemon juice – this will help release more minerals into the broth.

Add pink Himalayan salt (whole or powdered). While adding vinegar to bone broth helps release the gelatin and minerals from the bones, pink Himalayan rock salt adds extra minerals, including potassium!

Pressure Cooker: Lock the lid of your pressure cooker and turn to high pressure / high heat. Once it reaches high pressure (either you have an indicator or in case of old pressure cookers, see a small amount of vapor escaping through the valve), turn to the lowest heat and set the timer for 90 minutes.

Dutch oven or Slow cooker: Cover with a lid and cook for at least 6 hours (high setting) or up to 10 hours (low setting). To release even more gelatine and minerals, you can cook it up to 48 hours. To do that, you'll have to remove the oxtail using thongs and shred the meat off using a fork. Then, you can place the bones back to the pot and cook up to 48 hours.

Pressure cooker: When done, take off heat and let the pressure release naturally for about 10-15 minutes. Remove the lid. Remove the large bits and pour the broth through a strainer into a large dish. Discard the vegetables and set the meaty bones aside to cool down.

When the meaty bones are chilled, shred the meat off the bone with a fork. If there is any gelatine left on the bones, you can reuse the bones again for another batch of bone broth. Just keep in the freezer and add some new pieces when making bone broth again. Use the juicy oxtail meat in other recipes (on top of lettuce leaves, with cauli-rice or as omelet filling) or eat with some warm bone broth.

Use the broth immediately or place in the fridge overnight, where the broth will become jelly. Oxtail is high in fat and the greasy layer on top (tallow) will solidify. Simply scrape most of the tallow off (as much as you wish).

Keep the broth in the fridge if you are planning to use it over the next 5 days. For future uses, place in small containers and freeze.

347. Faux Paleo Napoleon

Ingredients:
Dough:
2 ½ cups almond flour
½ teaspoon baking soda
¼ teaspoon sea salt
½ cup + 2 tablespoons organic palm shortening, slightly melted so that it's easy to mix
2 tablespoons honey
1 tablespoon vanilla extract
Filling:
2 cups almond flour
½ cup organic palm shortening or butter (I used shortening. Can't vouch for the results if butter is used, but I don't see why it wouldn't work.)
¼ cup honey
1 tablespoon vanilla extract
⅛ teaspoon sea salt
1 cup chopped fruit of choice for topping
Instruction:
Preheat oven to 325 degrees.
Mix all of the dry dough ingredients in a large bowl. Then add in all of the wet dough ingredients. Stir to combine.
Move dough to a silicone baking mat or parchment paper, and roll it out with a rolling pin or something similar. If you need to use your hands, make sure you wet them with water first so that the dough doesn't stick to you.
Using a pastry cutter, cut the dough into 12 equal-sized squares (or rectangles) about 3 (or 2.5) inches wide and 3 inches tall. No need to pull them apart. Once they're done baking, if you can't get them apart easily, just use the pastry cutter again to separate them.
Carefully transfer the baking mat or parchment paper (with the dough on it) to a baking sheet.
Bake for about 10-15 minutes, or until the dough is cooked through and a little bit crispy (like a pie crust would be).
Mix all of the filling ingredients together, except for the fruit.
Once the dough has cooled you can put your layers together. Layer a piece of dough, about 3-4 tablespoons of filling (spread it out), a piece of dough, more filling, a piece of dough, more filling, then some cherries.
Begin a new one. Do this until you run out of dough and filling.

348. Fish Fillet Delux

Ingredients:
4 white fish fillets, about 5 oz each
4 tsp olive oil
Low sodium salt and fresh pepper, to taste
4 sprigs fresh herbs (parsley, rosemary, oregano)
1 lemon, sliced thin
4 large pieces heavy duty aluminum foil,
Instructions:
Place the fish in the center of the foil, season with low sodium salt and pepper and drizzle with olive oil. Place a slice of lemon on top of each piece of fish, then a sprig of herbs on each. Fold up the edges so that it's completely sealed and no steam will escape, creating a loose tent.
Heat half of the grill (on one side) on high heat with the cover closed. When the grill is hot, place the foil packets on the side of the grill with the burners off (indirect heat) and close the grill. Depending on the thickness of your fish, cook 10 to 15 minutes, or until the fish is opaque and cooked through.....serve with green salad and paleo dressing.

349. Roasted Paleo Citrus and Herb Chicken

Ingredients
12 total pieces bone-in chicken thighs and legs
1 medium onion, thinly sliced
1 tbsp dried rosemary
1 tsp dried thyme
1 lemon, sliced thin
1 orange, sliced thin
For the marinade
5 tbsp extra virgin olive oil
6 cloves garlic, minced
1 tbsp honey
Juice of 1 lemon
Juice of 1 orange
1 tbsp Italian seasoning
1 tsp onion powder
Dash of red pepper flakes
Salt and freshly ground pepper, to taste
Instructions
Whisk together all of the marinade ingredients in a small bowl. Place the chicken in a baking dish (or a large Ziploc bag) and pour the marinade over it. Marinate for 3 hours to overnight.
Preheat the oven to 400 degrees F. Place the chicken in a baking dish and arrange with the onion, orange, and lemon slices. Sprinkle with thyme, rosemary, salt and pepper. Cover with aluminum foil and bake for 30 minutes. Remove the foil, baste the chicken, and bake for another 30 minutes uncovered, until the chicken is cooked through.
Notes
Servings: 4-6
Difficulty: Easy

350. Stove-top "Cheesy" Paleo Chicken Casserole

Ingredients
2 cups shredded cooked chicken
1 1/2 cups cooked butternut squash (about 1 small squash)
1/2 cup coconut cream, skimmed from the top of a can of coconut milk
1/4 cup coconut oil, melted
1 heaping cup green peas, thawed
1 tbsp apple cider vinegar
1/2 tsp salt
1/2 tsp oregano
1/2 tsp thyme
1 tbsp fresh parsley, for garnish
Instructions
In a large bowl, mash the butternut squash. Stir in the coconut cream, oil, vinegar, salt, oregano, and thyme. Once everything is combined, add in the shredded chicken and peas.
Place the mixture into a large saucepan and cook over medium heat for 5-8 minutes, until the peas are cooked and squash is creamy. Top with fresh parsley and serve warm.
Notes
Servings: 4-5
Difficulty: Medium

351. Homemade Herbed Paleo Mayonnaise

Ingredients
1 egg (at room temperature)
2 tbsp lemon juice
1 tsp rosemary
1 tsp oregano
½ tsp sea salt
1 cup light olive oil (not EVOO – the flavour will be too strong)
This recipe will make approximately 24 1tbsp servings

Directions
Add egg, lemon juice, rosemary, oregano, and sea salt to a mixing bowl.
Whisk together with an electric mixer on low until well blended. Don't turn off the mixer at any point during this process. While still whisking, slowly add in your olive oil. Slow is the key word here. Like, one little drizzle at a time slow. Slowly but surely, you'll see the emulsion start to form. Once you see the emulsion forming, continue to add in your olive oil just as slowly until your mayonnaise reaches the desired consistency.
Refrigerate in a glass jar and enjoy! Will last in the fridge approximately one week.

Nutrition Facts Per Serving
Calories: 56
Total Fat: 6.5g
Saturated Fat: 1.0g
Carbs: 0.1g
Protein: 0.2g

352. Homemade Paleo Ketchup with a Kick

Ingredients
1 12 oz can tomato paste
1 cup water
2 tbsp vinegar
½ tsp salt
½ tsp curry powder
½ tsp garlic powder
This recipe makes approximately 32 oz of ketchup, or 64 1tbsp servings.
Directions
Mix all ingredients in a sauce pan and bring to boil on medium-high heat.
Reduce heat to medium-low and simmer while stirring frequently until flavours have blended. (Add more water for thinner ketchup, add less water for thicker)
Transfer to a glass jar and cool before serving.
Nutrition Facts Per Serving
Calories: 5
Total Fat: 0.0g
Sodium: 21mg
Carbs: 1.0g
Protein: 0.7g

353. Homemade Paleo Honey Mustard from Scratch

Ingredients
1/4 cup mustard powder
1/4 cup water
3 tbsp honey
Sea salt, to taste
Instructions
Place the mustard powder and water in a bowl and stir until combined. Add salt and honey to taste. Let stand for at least 15 minutes before serving.
Notes
Servings: about 1/2 cup
Difficulty: Easy

354. All-Natural Homemade Paleo Apple Butter

Ingredients
5 apples, peeled, cored and diced
2/3 cup apple cider
1/3 cup honey
1 tbsp cinnamon
1/2 tsp salt
Pinch of cloves, optional

Instructions
Place all of the ingredients into the slow cooker and stir to evenly coat. Cover and cook on low heat for 6 hours. Let cool slightly and puree in a food processor or blender until smooth.

Notes
Servings: 4-6
Difficulty: Easy

355. Homemade Paleo BBQ Sauce (YUM)

Ingredients
15 oz. organic tomato sauce
1 cup water
1/2 cup apple cider vinegar
1/3 cup honey
1 tbsp lemon juice
2 tsp onion powder
1 1/2 tsp ground black pepper
1 1/2 tsp ground mustard
1 tsp paprika
Instructions
Combine all of the ingredients in a medium saucepan over medium-high heat. Stir to combine. Bring to a boil, and then reduce to simmer for 1 hour. Taste and adjust seasonings as desired. Serve with meat or store in an airtight container in the refrigerator.
Notes
Servings: about 1 1/2 cups
Difficulty: Easy

356. Basil Pesto

Ingredients
1 large bunch of basil (approx. 2 cups)
1/3 cup walnuts or pine nuts
2 medium garlic cloves, minced
1/2 cup Parmigiano Reggiano or other Parmesan cheese (optional)
approx. 1/3 cup extra virgin olive oil
salt and pepper to taste

Instructions
Place basil, nuts, garlic and cheese (optional) in food processor.
Run the food processor, pausing to add olive oil to reach desired consistency.
Salt and pepper to taste.

357. Paleo Chicken Tortilla Soup

Ingredients
2 large chicken breasts, skin removed and cut into ½ inch strips
1 28oz can of diced tomatoes
32 ounces organic chicken broth
1 sweet onion, diced
2 jalepenos, de-seeded and diced
2 cups of shredded carrots
2 cups chopped celery
1 bunch of cilantro chopped fine
4 cloves of garlic, minced - I always use one of these
2 Tbs tomato paste
1 tsp chili powder
1 tsp cumin
sea salt & fresh cracked pepper to taste
olive oil
1-2 cups water

Instructions
In a crockpot or large dutch oven over med-high heat, place a dash of olive oil and about ¼ cup chicken broth. Add onions, garlic, jalapeno, sea salt and pepper and cook until soft, adding more broth as needed.
Then add all of your remaining ingredients and enough water to fill to the top of your pot. Cover and let cook on low for about 2 hrs, adjusting salt & pepper as needed.
Once the chicken is fully cooked, you should be able to shred it very easily. I simply used the back of a wooden spoon and pressed the cooked chicken against the side of the pot. You could also use a fork or tongs to break the chicken apart and into shreds.
Top with avocado slices and fresh cilantro. Enjoy!
This is an easy one-pot meal that's loaded with veggies, low in fat, and full of flavour! You don't need to add cheese or tortilla strips the soup is full of flavour on it's own!

358. Paleo Eggs Benedict on Artichoke Hearts

Eggs Benedict
4 eggs
1 egg white (use from Hollandaise Sauce Recipe below)
250 grams of bacon
4 Artichoke Hearts
3/4 cup of balsamic vinegar
salt and pepper to taste
Hollandaise Sauce
4 egg yolks
1 tbsp of lemon juice
pinch of salt and paprika
¾ cup of melted ghee

Directions

Line a baking sheet with foil and set aside. Preheat your oven to 375 degrees. Deconstruct your artichokes and remove the artichoke hearts. Place the hearts in balsamic vinegar for 20 minutes.

For your Hollandaise Sauce, place a pot of water to simmer on your stove. Melt the ghee in a saucepan. Separate your eggs and place the yolks in a stainless steel cooking bowl. Hold on to the egg whites for the next step.

Remove your hearts from the marinade and place on cookie sheet, brush the tops of them with the egg white and then place your bacon over the artichokes as a second layer. Stick your tray in the oven for 20 minutes.

Back to the sauce, whisk the yolks with the lemon juice and then place your bowl over the simmering water. Slowly add in the ghee and bit of salt and continue to whisk until your sauce doubles in size and is silky. Set aside.

To poach your eggs, turn up the heat on your stove and let the same water get to a rolling boil. Crack your eggs one at a time into a ladle and the slide the egg into the water. Give them about a minute and a half and remove.

Now you are ready to assemble. Grab your artichoke hearts and bacon, then lay your poached egg and pour the Hollandaise silk on top.

359. Hearty Paleo Jambalaya

Ingredients
1 tbsp extra virgin olive oil
8 oz. Andouille sausage, diced
1/2 red bell pepper, diced
1/2 yellow bell pepper, diced
4 cloves garlic, minced
1/2 medium onion, diced
1 14.5-oz. can fire-roasted tomatoes
1 tbsp smoked paprika
1 tsp dried thyme
1 tsp cumin
Dash of cayenne pepper
1 1/2 cups chicken broth
1 large head of cauliflower, coarsely chopped
1 lb. medium shrimp, peeled and deveined
Salt and pepper, to taste
Fresh cilantro, for garnish

Instructions
Heat the olive oil in a Dutch oven or heavy-bottomed saucepan. Add the Andouille sausages and cook for 4-5 minutes until lightly browned. Add the red and yellow peppers, garlic, and onion and stir. Cook for 4 minutes until softened.
Stir in the tomatoes and spices. Pour in the chicken stock and bring to a boil. Once boiling, turn the heat down and simmer for 20 minutes.
Meanwhile, place the cauliflower into a food processor and pulse until it is reduced to the size of rice grains.
Mix in the cauliflower rice to the jambalaya, starting with half of the rice and adding more depending on preference. Simmer for 12-15 minutes until tender. Add the shrimp and cook everything for 5-7 minutes until the shrimp are opaque. Season to taste with salt and pepper. Serve hot, garnished with fresh cilantro.

Notes
Servings: 4-6
Difficulty: Easy

Paleo Diet Recipes 365 Days of Paleo and Coconut Recipes by Mercedes Del Rey

360. Shrimp & Grits (Paleo Style)

For the shrimp
15 pieces raw shrimp, shelled and de-veined
3 tbsp extra virgin olive oil
6 garlic cloves minced, divided
Zest from one lemon
2 tsp dried oregano, divided
2 slices bacon
1/2 large onion, diced
2 tbsp butter
1 tbsp white wine vinegar
1 tsp red pepper flakes
1 tbsp lemon juice
1 tbsp chopped fresh oregano
Salt and freshly ground black pepper, to taste
For the grits
1 large head of cauliflower, cut into florets
1/4 cup almond milk
4 garlic cloves, minced
1 tbsp ghee or butter
1/4 tsp cayenne pepper
Salt and pepper, to taste
Instructions
In a medium bowl mix together the olive oil, 2 cloves of garlic, lemon zest, and 1 teaspoon dried oregano. Place shrimp in the bowl and marinate for 1-3 hours.

Place a couple inches of water in a large pot. Once water is boiling, place steamer insert and then cauliflower florets into the pot and cover. Steam for 12-14 minutes, until completely tender. Drain and return cauliflower to pot.

Add the milk, ghee, and garlic to the cauliflower. Using an immersion blender, combine ingredients. The cauliflower should be fairly thick to resemble the consistency of grits. Season with salt and pepper to taste.

Cook the bacon in a large skillet over medium heat until crispy. Reserving the bacon fat in the pan, set the bacon aside to cool and break into pieces.

Add the butter to the bacon fat in the pan and melt. Add the onion and sauté for 4-5 minutes until softened. Add in the remaining 4 garlic cloves, dried oregano, and the red pepper flakes. Sauté for 1-2 minutes, stirring frequently.

Stir in the white wine vinegar, and then add the shrimp. Cook, stirring frequently, until the shrimp are cooked through, 3-4 minutes. Remove from heat and stir in the lemon juice. Season with salt and pepper. Serve shrimp and onions over grits, with bacon and fresh oregano for garnish.

Notes
Servings: 3-4
Difficulty: Medium

361. How to Make Paleo Cauliflower "Rice"

Ingredients
1 head of cauliflower
½ Vidalia onion
3 cloves of garlic
1 tbsp coconut oil
salt and pepper, to taste
This recipe makes 2-3 servings, depending on the size of your cauliflower.
Instructions
Remove leaves and stem from cauliflower; discard. Grate the entire head of cauliflower until it resembles rice.
Dice the onions and garlic to your desired size.
Add coconut oil to a pan over medium heat. Add in onion and garlic until slightly browned.
Add in grated cauliflower, salt, and pepper and stir until heated.

362. Paleo Cocoa Puffs

Ingredients
¾ Packed Cup of Blanched Almond Flour
1 Cup + 2 Tbsp Tapioca Starch/Flour
½ Cup Cocoa Powder
¼ tsp Salt
⅔ cup Coconut Palm Sugar
2½ tsp. Baking Powder
1 Tbsp Vanilla Extract
⅓ Cup of oil or Melted Butter (dairy or nondairy)
1 Egg + 1 Egg White

Instructions
Preheat Oven to 350 degrees.
Mix together the dry ingredients (Almond Flour, Tapioca Flour, Cocoa Powder, Salt, Palm Sugar, and Baking Powder).
Add in the Vanilla, Oil, and Eggs. Mix really well (don't be afraid to get your hands dirty!)
Line 2 large baking sheets with parchment paper.
Roll teaspoon sized balls of dough (or smaller if you have the patience) in between your palms to create little cocoa puff balls. If you find your hands getting sticky- rinse them off and dry them before continuing and or dust your hands with a little extra tapioca starch.
Use about half the dough to make cocoa puffs for the first baking sheet. Leave a little space between each cocoa puff as they will expand in the oven.
Place the first baking sheet into the oven and bake 18-20 minute. Halfway through baking using a spatula to flip the cocoa puffs over so that the bottoms do not burn.
While the first tray is baking, prepare your second tray of cocoa puffs and follow the same baking instructions.
Let cocoa puffs cool completely before eating. (They will get crispy as they cool).

363. Tantalizing Prawn Skewers

Ingredients:
1 lb jumbo raw tiger prawns, shelled and deveined (weight after peeled)
2 cloves garlic, crushed
Low sodium salt and pepper
8 long wooden skewers

Instructions:
Soak the skewers in water at least 20 minutes to prevent them from burning.

Combine the prawns with crushed garlic and season with low sodium salt and pepper. You can let this marinate for a while, or even overnight.

Heat a clean, lightly oiled grill to medium heat, when the grill is hot add the prawns, careful not to burn the skewers. Grill on both sides for about 6 - 8 minutes total cooking time or until the prawns are opaque and cooked through.

Squeeze lemon juice over the prawns and serve with green salad and my paleo dressing

364. Paleo BLT Frittata

Ingredients
8 eggs
4 slices bacon, cooked and chopped
3-4 cups spinach (or other greens of your choice)
1 large tomato, sliced and seeded
1 tbsp almond milk
1/2 tsp salt
1/4 tsp pepper
2 tbsp chopped fresh basil
1 tbsp extra virgin olive oil

Instructions

Preheat oven to 400 degrees F. In a medium bowl, whisk together the eggs, milk, basil, salt and pepper. Set aside.

Heat olive oil in a 10-inch nonstick skillet over medium heat. Add greens and cook 3-4 minutes until wilted. Add in bacon and stir.

Add egg mixture to the pan and place tomatoes on top. Using a spatula, occasionally lift the edges to allow uncooked egg to run under. When the frittata has set, transfer to the oven and cook for 12-15 minutes or until egg is cooked through. Cut into wedges and serve warm.

Notes
Servings: 5
Difficulty: Easy

365. Extra Easy Broth

Ingredients
4 - 8 lbs of bones, from grass fed animals (depending on the size of stock pot)
2 Tbsp apple cider vinegar
vegetables, carrots, onions, celery
water

Instructions

Roast the bones in the oven at 375 F for 1 hour. This gives a good flavour to the stock.

Remove the bones from the oven and place in a stock pot.

Fill the pot with water - cover the bones.

Add the vegetables - avoid Brussels sprouts, cabbage, broccoli, turnips as these tend to give a bitter flavour to the broth.

Bring the water to a boil and add the vinegar.

Turn the pot down to a simmer.

Allow the broth to simmer for 24 hours or longer.

As it cooks, add water as necessary and skim off any foam.

When finished, strain the broth through a wire mesh and catch the broth in mason jars.

Once cooled, the fat will rise to the top and the broth should gel like gelatine.

The fat can be skimmed off and used for cooking or left in the broth.

The broth will keep refrigerated for 1 week and can also be frozen for months.

Paleo Diet Recipes 365 Days of Paleo and Coconut Recipes by Mercedes Del Rey

About The Author

If you're a sufferer from any kind of immune deficiency disorder, I especially want to extend a warm welcome to you. Welcome, my friend, to my wonderful world of completely safe and natural healing. My name is Mercedes del Rey but my friends and patients call me Merche and I am truly fortunate to live in one of the most beautiful places in the world. My home is in sunny Andalusia in the south of Spain, the place where I was born and where I grew up before travelling to the US to complete my higher education. My life has been blessed in so many ways but, like so many people, I've also had to contend with plenty of problems along the way.

Despite growing up in such a wonderful place, my health has not always been very strong. For example, my immune system was a constant source of worry and I suffered from a series of acute and often debilitating allergies throughout my childhood, sometimes reacting to certain foods and then to the chemicals in ordinary household articles like hand soap and shampoo. I seemed to pick every bug and infection that was going round. A deficient immune system can do that. Eventually, the conditions became severe and I began my long exposure to the medical profession and a cocktail of drugs that were supposed to balance my immune system and calm my allergies but, in the end, they only succeeded in making my life more miserable because of all the unpleasant side effects. Doctors rarely mention the negative consequences of the drugs they prescribe but I could see that my condition was becoming worse rather than getting better.

There were times when I suffered from bouts of depression and a complete lack of confidence, always conscious of the rashes and the embarrassing marks on my skin, the unexplained outbreaks of eczema and the fear of being disfigured by the horrible patches that appeared on my face and body. Sometimes it seemed that my immune system was attacking me rather than protecting me. In some ways, growing up was a nightmare. Like so many other unhappy people, I turned to food as a source of comfort and then I started to gain weight, which made me feel even worse! I was highly strung, super-sensitive, borderline depressed and often miserable. The drugs were no help whatsoever. The fact is that my immune system had been further compromised by the constant stream of allergies and by the medication that had been prescribed for my various conditions. And then, as if out of the blue, I met someone who turned my life around completely.

A friend was very concerned about me. She knew I wasn't sleeping well, that my allergies were a constant source of discomfort and embarrassment, that I was depressed and that I'd hit a low spot in my life where i no longer knew where to turn for help. She recommended someone to me, a very special person, a lady who understood exactly what was wrong with me and who showed me how to change my life forever using the most natural remedies imaginable. Her name is Beran Parry and her knowledge of herbalism opened my life to an extraordinary world of natural healing. Beran has a very wide knowledge and experience of health, nutrition and all the factors that can contribute to complete wellbeing. The results of her advice and guidance were simply astonishing. My allergies and

Paleo Diet Recipes 365 Days of Paleo and Coconut Recipes by Mercedes Del Rey

have disappeared and my immune system is functioning perfectly. I don't even get colds or 'flu anymore, and that in itself is quite remarkable! My mood swings have vanished. I sleep wonderfully and my confidence has soared. I was so impressed by her knowledge and passion for natural healing that I became her pupil and studied with her for several years. She has inspired me to travel the world on my quest to research and investigate herbal medicine and all that it entails.

I visited China, India, Germany, the USA and Canada and met with so many wonderful Naturopathic Doctors and Herbalists along my learning path.

I now practice as a Holistic Nutritionist and I advise my own clients on the use and application of herbal remedies. It was Beran, of course, who encouraged me to write this book and she assisted me with my research and studies. My dearest hope is that it proves to be as useful and helpful to you as her teaching has been to me.

This is not a medical advice book so please always check any remedy with your medical and naturopathic doctor at all times!

May the force of Nature be with you!

Paleo Diet Recipes 365 Days of Paleo and Coconut Recipes by Mercedes Del Rey

DOWNLOAD YOUR FREE PALEO EPIGENETIC DIET EBOOK

AND START LOSING WEIGHT TODAY

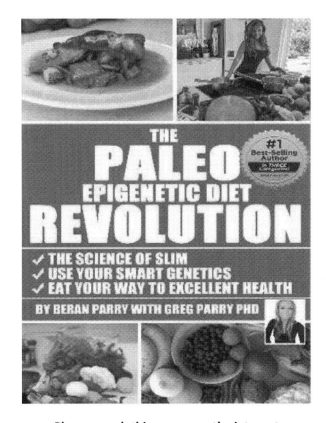

Please search this page over the internet
www.skinnydeliciouslife.com/free-epigenetic-diet-ebook

Paleo Diet Recipes 365 Days of Paleo and Coconut Recipes by Mercedes Del Rey

Before You Go.......

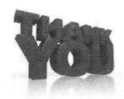

I am so delighted that you have chosen this book and it's been a pleasure writing it for you. My mission is to help as many readers as possible to benefit from the content you have just been reading. So many of us are able to take new information and apply it to our lives with really positive and long lasting consequences and it is my wish that you have been able to take value from the information I have presented.

Thank you for staying with me during this book and for reading it through to the end. I really hope that you have enjoyed the contents and that's why I appreciate your feedback so much. If you could take a couple of minutes to review the book, your views will help me to create more material that you find beneficial.

I am always thrilled to hear from my readers and you can email me personally via the publisher at beranparry@gmail.com if you have any questions about this book or future books. Let us know how we can help you by sending a message to the same email address.

Thanks again for your support and encouragement. I really look forward to reading your review.

Please go to the book product page to complete your review

Stay Healthy!

Paleo Diet Recipes 365 Days of Paleo and Coconut Recipes by Mercedes Del Rey

FOR MORE BY

MERCEDES DEL REY

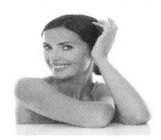

Please search this page over the www.amazon.com amzn.to/2kSzZnU

Manufactured by Amazon.ca
Bolton, ON

29869313R10216